CARE
for the CARER

AN ALZHEIMER'S MEMOIR

Jeff Camhi

Other books
by Jeff Camhi

*Neuroethology: Nerve Cells and the
Natural Behavior of Animals*

*A Dam in the River: Releasing the
Flow of University Ideas*

Fifty Tree Tales
(co-authored with Michael Avishai)

CONTENTS

Acknowledgments

Many thanks to Ilana Blumberg, Judy Labensohn, Ilene Prusher, Barbara Gingold, Nadia Jacobson, Nikki Littman, and the Laura of this book for welcoming me into creative nonfiction writing with courses, workshops, editing, and encouragement; to members of my writer's group, especially June Levitt, Judy Cardozo, Bill Taeusch, and Reva Mann; to my sons, Jeremy and Alon, for their feedback and encouragement; and to my late wife, Jane, for having encouraged my writing even before I began typing out our lives.

A portion of this book was published in a slightly different form in the *Michigan Quarterly Review* (2018).

When my advisor asked me, "Why don't you take yourself away, maybe to a beachside hotel for a few days?" I didn't understand how she could suggest such a thing. Who would take care of Jane? How could I enjoy myself, not knowing if she was okay? I would probably feel even worse at the beach than right there in our home.

PART I

JANE AND JEFF

|1|

Through the Window

One Sunday morning in September 1963 in my ground-floor rental in Cambridge, Massachusetts, a book about how the brain functions had me riveted. Then someone tapped on my window, breaking my concentration. A woman called in through the dusty glass and the venetian blind. "Excuse me. Someone told me there's an apartment for rent here. Is that right?" Inserting a pencil to hold my page, I pointed toward the front door and stepped into the lobby to meet her: thin-waisted, sunglasses propped on her curly black hair, turtleneck tucked into tight black pants, a small notepad in one hand, a lit cigarette in the other.

I explained that there were six small apartments in the house, and a guy upstairs had recently finished his studies and moved out.

The building manager had announced that the apartment was now available at the same low monthly rent as mine.

"You a student here?" I asked.

She exhaled smoke over her shoulder. "No, post-MA and taking a break."

She was planning on a doctorate, she explained, but first needed to earn some cash. Would it be okay for her to live there though she wasn't a student?

It was a university-owned building, and most residents, like me, were first-year PhD students. Yet it was open to all, I told her, already imagining her as one of the all. The vacant apartment was unlocked, and I suggested she go up and have a look.

She bolted up the stairs and then quickly bounced back down. "I'll give that manager a yes," she exclaimed, tucking her notepad into her pocket. "Never thought getting into Harvard would be this easy!"

She reached a hand toward mine. "I'm Jane."

Firm grip, I noted.

"Jeff," I replied.

She moved into the upstairs apartment two days later. I thought it appropriate to invite her to my place for dinner.

* * *

A jazz LP blasted out from my hi-fi as burgers grilled, onions sizzled, and Heinz cream of tomato soup bubbled away in the open kitchen. Jane helped me move my wobbly table and two wicker chairs away from their crowded corner.

She pointed to the wooden desk by my window.

"Let me guess—you built that yourself, right? I did that too, in my Berkeley apartment—a wooden door, some two-by-fours, a few nails, and you're officially a grad student, right?"

She had done her MA in medieval history, she explained, and then came east, partly "to breathe in the Ivy League air." Also, having no siblings, she wanted to be closer to her parents. They had moved some years before to Manhattan from upstate New York—the little town of Saranac Lake, right in the middle of the Adirondack Mountains, where Jane had grown up.

"Not exactly the Himalayas," she confessed, "but high enough to get my blood pumping on weekend climbs." She had climbed forty different Adirondack peaks, she asserted, before graduating high school.

Her parents had moved to Saranac Lake when Jane was in grade school so her father could be treated for his tuberculosis at the famous Trudeau Institute. His illness had changed their lives, she explained. It made Jane's mother his nearly full-time carer and Jane herself a kind of substitute carer, although she was permitted to be with him only ten minutes a day, with no touching, out on the covered but open porch where he spent his days and nights, even throughout the harsh Adirondack winters—all part of his treatment.

In her teens, Jane mirrored her mother by playing the role of carer with her close friends, getting them all to exercise together and even trying out her own teenage version of psychoanalysis on them. She particularly looked after one friend, a boy who was in a wheelchair.

As I ladled the soup, Jane pulled off her sandals and dug her feet into the carpet, its white wool wisps twisting around her toes.

"Who's that tooting the sax on your hi-fi?" she asked.

"Trumpet. That's Miles."

"As in 'miles to go before he sleeps?'"

"As in Davis. He's the greatest; the man's got soul."

"Sounds like you know something about music," she remarked as we settled into our chairs. "And maybe about soul?"

She was right about music. I'd started classical piano lessons when I was six, I told her, though they didn't interest me much until I was around twelve. Then I'd practice for my own sake, not my teacher's, going over and over some Mozart or Beethoven phrase until I got it exactly as *I* wanted it. "But jazz was waiting in the wings," I said. "At around age fifteen, I moved into improvisation and never left it." I so wished I'd had my baby grand at that moment—I'd play Jane a few of my favorite songs. But there was no room for it in my cramped apartment. When I moved to a bigger place, my parents would surely ship it to me.

"Listen to what Miles does next." I pointed to the hi-fi speaker.

He spun a happy phrase around, and it came out so mournful it almost hurt. Jane didn't comment. Instead she asked, "Do you know 'Love Is Like a Cigarette'?"

"No, how exactly is love like that?"

"It's the title of a song. My father wrote it—well, the lyrics, anyway—and lots of other songs, too. Duke Edgington recorded that one," she added with a nonchalant backward sweep of her hand.

"You mean Ellington? Wow, really?"

She scanned my LP collection. "Do you have any Dylan? Like 'Blowin' in the Wind'? He really gets it, you know," she said.

I shook my head. Not my kind of music, I explained.

She asked if I'd been to the Lincoln Memorial the previous month to hear King's "I Have a Dream" speech; she could kick herself, she said, for not having been there.

I had never actually thought of being there, I explained, though I would never forget the depth, the power, the beauty of the speech, which I'd heard on the radio.

"What moves me most, though, is *The Feminine Mystique*," Jane continued. I must have looked blank. "You know, Betty Friedan's new book. Women's new voice."

I pointed to the book on my desk about the brain and told her that was what moved me the most. "The author claims that those three-pound lumps of tissue inside your skull and mine and everyone else's are the most complex objects in the world."

Jane knocked her knuckles against her

forehead and whispered, with a nervous laugh, "Not so sure about that."

"Oh, I think he's right, and I hope that someday I can help figure out how all that complexity works."

I twisted the cork out of a cheap bottle of Chianti, apologizing that it was all I could afford on my doctoral fellowship, and brought in a plate of saltine crackers I'd spread with cream cheese and powdered with paprika.

Sipping her Chianti, she commented, "If you want to know about cheap wine, it was that sugary kosher stuff I grew up drinking every Friday night with my parents."

It hadn't occurred to me she might be Jewish. Nice to know, though. Not only Jewish, it turned out her parents kept a kosher home, and she even had some Orthodox cousins. She mentioned several Jewish history courses she'd taken at Berkeley and a job she'd had earlier, while at Barnard, helping a professor research medieval Jewish migrations.

Back then, she said, she'd wanted to make a Jewish migration of her own. She picked up a cracker and dug her knife into the cream cheese at one corner, explaining, "I would start right here, in America," then she gouged a direct route to the cracker's far corner, "and I'd fly all the way over here to Israel." Her plan had been to study agriculture and make the desert bloom. But then she decided to put all that on hold.

"How come?"

"Boyfriend. Not Jewish."

"Ahh."

She broke off a piece of cracker, placed it in her mouth, and crunched. "The Israel idea went *poof*," she said as little flecks of cracker flew from her lips, and we both laughed.

"And the boyfriend?"

"Also *poof*," she said, this time lifting a hand in front of her mouth.

I couldn't imagine why she would have even thought of giving up on America for Israel. I mentioned how, during college, my father had pushed me to apply for a summer job there at the Weizmann Institute. A friend of his could recommend me. It seemed weird, I explained, because in our house we hardly ever talked about Israel or even about being Jewish. Of course, I'd had a bar mitzvah, but it meant little to me except that everyone seemed happy and I got lots of presents.

"So did you ever actually go to Israel?" she asked.

"Hell, no. I was a spoiled kid from the New York suburbs. Hastings-on-Hudson, if you please. Pioneering in the desert? You maybe, but not me."

Looking around my room, Jane spotted my tennis racket and asked if I did any regular exercise.

I gave that a negative.

She had the Royal Canadian Mounted Police book of exercises and did their workout early every morning. Would I like to join her? It would be good for me, she suggested.

But I was busy organizing the dessert. I had gone out on a limb with fried bananas and ice cream. "Do you prefer yours with vanilla or chocolate?"

"How would I know?" she asked. "Six o'clock tomorrow. Exercise. Okay for you?"

"Not really, and are you telling me you've never had ice cream with your fried bananas?" I asked.

"Nor fried bananas minus ice cream," she replied, and declared, "Six o'clock it is, then."

In the end, she chose chocolate, I vanilla.

A bridgeable divide, I told myself.

Like medieval history and brain science.

* * *

A knock on my apartment door woke me. I checked the time—six o'clock.

"Yeah?"

"It's me. Exercise time," Jane called out.

"Not really." I fell back to sleep.

Next morning, six o'clock, another knock.

"Go away."

"Not really," she replied.

Silence.

Then shuffling noises on the porch just outside my window.

The scraping sound of the window sliding open.

Rustling of the venetian blind.

Lying cheek on pillow, I soon spied next to my bed two bare feet digging into the floppy wisps of my carpet. A tug on my pajama sleeve encouraged me out of bed, so I strode to my dresser, grabbed a handful of clothes, disappeared into the bathroom, and emerged dressed and wondering what tortures she and the Royal Mounted Police had in store for me.

"On your back, we start with legs—lift and hold," she directed, lying down beside me on the carpet.

I managed to hold mine a few inches off the floor for the better part of a minute. So did Jane. But while my stomach muscles trembled at Richter nine, hers held steady as Gibraltar. These were followed by sit-ups, push-ups, and other tortures. It went on for half an hour.

"I hate the Royal Mounted Police!" I groaned.

Jane scheduled us for the same time the next morning, turned the latch to open my door, suggested I might want to leave it unlocked on subsequent nights, and was gone.

Our morning exercises became a daily routine.

Sometimes we touched.

* * *

We slid toward couplehood, with morning exercises, evening dinners at her place or mine, and ultimately, sleepovers. That continued right through my first Harvard year. Then that summer, I was to be away, taking a two-month course on modern experimental methods in neurobiology at the Marine Biological Laboratory in Woods Hole on Cape Cod. It was about an hour-and-a-half drive south of Cambridge, and I drove back for occasional weekends with Jane. I also phoned her a few times a week.

The day after I returned from one of my Cambridge visits, I was surprised by her phoning me.

She started the conversation with "I'm pregnant."

"I'm coming," I replied.

I hopped into my car and trembled most of the way north. Some impulse led me to drive about twenty minutes beyond Cambridge, to Tufts, my undergrad university. There, I headed for the music building and a specific piano practice room I knew well. I kept the ceiling lights low, placed my jittery hands on the keyboard, and began improvising on some doleful melodies. After an hour, I had managed to play most of the jitters out of me and felt ready, more or less, to meet Jane, though I had no idea how that meeting would go.

I pulled myself up the stairs to her apartment, knocked on her door, and hugged her tight in the doorway.

She didn't seem jittery, almost as though nothing much had happened.

She made coffee.

"We have two options," she stated, matter-of-factly. "Either we get married, or we don't and I raise the kid alone. I'm for the latter option."

I hadn't even thought about options, but I knew one thing right away and I knew it for sure—she was not going to "raise the kid alone." I had no idea where my certainty, my sudden confidence, came from; I just knew we were together and we were staying together, and as I told her that, I knew it was right.

I didn't make it down on one knee with a "Will you marry me?" proposal. It was more a matter of, "Here's the plan."

Jane looked surprised at my certainty, but also pleased. She chose to go with the plan.

All I could say was, "Good choice, Mom."

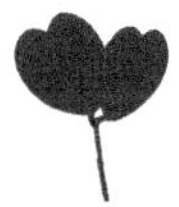

<| 2 |</p>

Family Support

Imagining that our plan might not go over so well with our parents, we decided not to tell them yet. Meanwhile, Jane looked for a justice of the peace. She chose an eighty-three-year-old Chinese Buddhist clergyman in Boston. Two weeks later, that spunky little man wrapped in a black robe picked up a rubber-tipped mallet and ceremoniously struck a giant brass gong that resonated through his spacious living room, proclaiming the start of our wedding. The only witness was the justice's much younger wife. Jane and I beamed right through the ceremony, which included his final, heavily accented blessing: "Love each other for what you are and forgive each other for what you ain't." At the word "ain't," he gave a little giggle.

We couldn't have known then how many times over the coming decades we would call upon this simple but wise blessing, printed below a photo of the two of us on a fridge magnet.

We did tell one couple about the wedding—our best friends, Cy and his wife, also named Jane. We'd wanted them to attend, but she was recovering from surgery in a Cambridge hospital. Cambridge was outside the justice's legal jurisdiction, but at his suggestion, right after the wedding, the three of us piled into my Chevy jalopy and headed for the other Jane's bedside. There, still wrapped in his black robe, the justice struck the porta-gong he'd brought along, setting alarmed nurses running into the room. A full, though unofficial, wedding ceremony followed, complete with—to the chagrin of the nurses—the throwing of rice. The two elderly patients who shared the room reached for their beds' control buttons, raised their backrests, and gawked.

* * *

Jane and I hadn't met each other's parents yet, and as we were now husband and wife, introductions seemed timely. We would remain silent, though, regarding our two weddings and the pregnancy.

We first visited Jane's parents in their Manhattan apartment. Although her father was hunched over and spoke with a wheeze, he greeted me with a vigorous handshake, flashed me a toothy smile, and dazzled me with wide-ranging, intelligent conversation. He certainly did not seem to be an invalid, though as Jane had explained to me, he had his good and his less-than-good days.

Curious about his songwriting, I asked how he had gotten started. He explained that he had majored in classics at Cornell before becoming a medical student at Columbia. But he quit medical school in his third year to become a songwriter. We shared a laugh when I divulged that I too had quit medical school—Yale in my case—and not during my third year, rather shortly after being accepted and before the studies had even begun, then switching to Harvard to become neither a doctor nor a song-writer but a neurobiologist. I sensed that he and I were going to get along well. During this conversation Jane's mother mostly sat, smiling quietly, her hands crossed on her lap, as if caring for her husband by yielding to him center stage.

Jane had told her dad that I played piano, though she herself had never heard me. He asked me to play something on their upright. How do you choose a song for your new in-laws who don't know that they're your in-laws? I simply selected a few of my Gershwin favorites and wove them together, drawing polite applause. Jane stepped up behind me and kissed the back of my head, as her father searched through some files on a bookshelf, pulled out the sheet music of his own song, "Love Is Like a Cigarette," and invited me to play it. I surprised him by saying, "Please don't expect me to live up to the Duke Ellington version."

When I finished, he applauded loudly and added, "The Duke's got nothing on you."

What a delightful first visit, I thought, already looking forward to many further occasions.

* * *

It was different when I took Jane to meet my parents, who had recently moved from the house where I'd grown up to an apartment in nearby Dobbs Ferry. My mom could no longer manage the long front stairway leading to our house.

Although I was sure that Jane and my mom would connect, I had my doubts about my father. Jane wasn't his type. She didn't do up her hair just so, dress in suburban fashion, or hold her tongue politely when she disagreed.

My father opened the door, and when I introduced Jane, he just pointed to the living room. Once there, I ran my hand smoothly, softly over the polished walnut wood of the baby grand piano. My mom tried to get up from the couch but couldn't manage it. I could see that her illness was advancing. I rushed to give her a big hug and kiss and then she and Jane embraced. Jane sat next to her, and soon the two were deep in conversation, as though they'd known each other for a long time. Jane told me later that, though she'd never before spoken with a cancer patient, she felt instantly comfortable with my mom.

My father, though, kept a cautious distance. He said little for the whole time we were there, holding his comments until I'd driven Jane to her parents' apartment and returned home for dinner.

At the table, he tore off a hunk of dinner roll, dunked it into a serving bowl, dredged out particles of vegetables and shrimp in olive oil, and plunged the entire mass into his mouth. A rivulet of oil trickled down his chin.

"She's a religious fanatic!" he began. "They've got a kosher home, for cryin' out loud. And she can't stop talking about Israel." He shook his head and drew his thumb across his chin, wiping off a fleck of shrimp.

I didn't answer.

"She's a radical socialist. Why is she so worried about all those black people and Puerto Ricans in New York without a dime in their pockets? Why don't they go out and work for a living like me?"

I struggled to remain quiet.

"You can bet one reason she's after you is my money."

I was starting to boil inside. He was talking about my wife. (Of course, he didn't know that.) Besides, would a "radical socialist" be after his money? My hand, under the table, was pinching my leg, telling me to remain silent.

"What is she, some kind of gypsy? Those … things she was wearing …"

Here my mom objected, saying that she liked Jane's outfit, in particular the bright, floral blouse and the several beaded necklaces. Not things she herself would wear, she added, but very attractive nonetheless. "I think she's a very nice girl, Meyer. And Jeff certainly seems to think so."

"What's the matter with you, Bea?" he snapped. "Can't you see? This girl's a parasite."

I struggled not to lash out at him, knowing that would only have made things worse. I'd learned that back in first or second grade when I started talking back to him. Then he would point his index finger just in front of my nose, poke his face forward, all knotted in anger, and whisper, "Don't you *dare* talk to your father like that!" He didn't touch my skin. Worse. He mauled my insides. That's when I developed a stutter. My mom took me to see a child psychologist every week for a year and then again in fifth or sixth grade. For both the stutter and the bed wetting.

Ever since then, when with him, I kept my thoughts mostly to myself. Now, for instance, I didn't tell him that I'd convinced Jane to quit the well-paying job she'd recently landed as administrative assistant to the head of a major printing company in Boston and instead enroll in a PhD program at Tufts in medieval history. Why would she work in business, which didn't interest her at all, when she could do what she loved in academia?

Were I to tell him this, he would probably have replied that "middle evil history," as he would likely pronounce it, was a waste of time. A woman, if she had to work, should be a schoolteacher or a nurse or maybe a secretary.

* * *

A few days later, Jane and I went for a long walk and decided to tell our parents that we had decided to get married and that we wanted a Jewish wedding soon, allowing us time for a brief honeymoon before the fall semester. Of course we didn't add that, within that brief time span, Jane would probably not yet be showing.

At the mention of a wedding, my mother glowed. My father scowled. The battle lines were drawn. Yet a small wedding was planned for just over a month hence in my parents' apartment.

Three days before the wedding, I was chatting with my older brother, Al, in my parents' apartment when the phone rang. My father answered. I could just about hear the wheezing, agitated voice of Jane's father, Jerome, on the line. I learned later that Jane had told him, perhaps unwisely, my father's opinions about how she dressed, how she spoke, what she believed.

Jerome yelled, "Let them go their own way!"

At first, my father didn't reply but finally argued that he had every right to say whatever he wanted to his son. He slammed the phone down and turned to me. "Well, your future father-in-law certainly has some nerve!"

Barely an hour later, the phone rang again, and I rushed to answer.

"Jeff, my father collapsed. It's awful. We're in Harlem Hospital."

"I'm coming."

In the emergency room, Jerome lay unconscious, wheezing shallow breaths into an oxygen mask. Tubes were everywhere. Jane's mother sat by his side, hunched over, eyes closed, her hands holding his, her lips whispering, perhaps praying.

Jane sat opposite her, softly stroking her dad's hair, her cheeks wet with tears. I stood beside her and kissed her hair. She held my hand.

The doctor arrived and sent us out to the hallway. Five minutes later he emerged: "I'm very sorry."

Jane and her mother clung to each other in silence. I placed a hand on Jane's shoulder, and she wrapped an arm around my waist. After some moments, Jane's mother lifted her hand and touched my arm. All she said was, "I couldn't do anything for him."

* * *

Following the funeral, attended by no one in my family but me, I wondered when we should reschedule the wedding. But Jane and her mother and, remarkably, my parents too, knew that, according to Jewish tradition, nothing delays a wedding. So we should pull ourselves together and, somehow, make room for a celebration—just days hence. I couldn't fathom how that would be possible.

Given the heaviness of all that had happened and sensing the need for a touch of levity, I asked Jane, "About not delaying a Jewish wedding, does that still apply when it's preceded by two Buddhist weddings, one of them in a hospital?"

I welcomed her smile.

On the wedding day, the rabbi, a family friend, was the first to arrive at my parents' apartment, even before Jane and her mother or any of the twenty or so guests. He sat with my father, Al and his wife, Ellen, and myself around my parents' bed, where my mom was resting to conserve her limited energy.

"Wait till you meet his girlfriend," my father sneered to the rabbi.

"You mean his bride, Meyer," my mother interjected.

He wrinkled his nose as though smelling something foul.

But the rabbi explained that Jane and I had come to see him, and we'd made "solid plans." He stressed that, as Jane was in mourning, we all needed to be especially kind to her. "And we need to help them both find their way."

"Find their way? I'll find my own way, thank you," my father replied. "Right out of here. Right now."

"Oh, Meyer" was all my mom could say. But strangely, as she did, she looked not at him, nor at me, but back and forth between Al and Ellen.

My father stood up. "I'm leaving now. I won't see my son married to *her*."

That was it! I shot up, glared straight at him, and declared, "It's too late for that. We're already married! We had a civil ceremony in Boston, nearly a month ago."

"You what?!" he roared.

"That's right. Shortly after we discovered that Jane's pregnant!"

"Meyer, a baby!" my mom gleamed.

My father lumbered toward me, his shoulders sagging, his arms dangling. "Well, you certainly made … these decisions … without … your parents." He plopped down on the bed. "Shame on you," he said, then repeated those three words several times.

He stayed for the wedding. But after the ceremony, as I was tasting the wedding cake, he approached me and advised, "Jeff, just remember—divorce is always an option." People near us heard and stared.

From that day on, my father never directed a single word to Jane. When we visited, he addressed only my mom and me as though Jane were absent. If he phoned us in Cambridge and Jane happened to answer, he would utter just three words: "Put Jeff on."

I felt torn in two. On the one hand, I wanted to honor my wife by refusing to visit my parents unless he started behaving properly. On the other hand, I knew that not visiting would hurt my mom. Jane tried as hard as she could to ignore him, but she occasionally broke into tears of sadness or anger or both.

* * *

In the early spring, I became a father. We named him Jeremy, after Jane's father, Jerome. I hoped to be a better father to Jeremy than my father had been to me. Jane, Jeremy, and I moved into a five-room, university-owned apartment near Harvard Yard. To my surprise and delight, my father shipped my piano to me with the note, "Now that you have more space, your mother says you should have this."

I was a second-year PhD student then and figured I would need about three more years to complete my doctorate. Then we would hopefully move to some university that would hire me, and I'd start my career of research and teaching. I was all of twenty-three years old but felt I was on my way.

| 3 |

There for Me

When I finished my PhD, Cornell University hired me as an assistant professor. We rented an apartment near the campus, in Ithaca, New York. Jane explored the Cornell library and found it rich in resources for her doctoral research. For Jeremy, we found an excellent day care arrangement nearby.

Jeremy and I enjoyed walks together around a small lake in the woods. We looked for beautiful little stones to take home, and we searched for crayfish under the rocks, which we would watch but leave alone. At home, we played with his model cars or made up games. When he was about five, we made up what became our favorite game. We called it Walnuts. We each had a stash of nuts, his shells marked with red dots, mine with blue, and we rolled them across the wooden living room floor, seeing who could get closest to a target we had placed there. It resembled British lawn bowls, except that we got down on our bellies to play.

I taught no courses of my own during my first year at Cornell but gave a few lectures in a group-taught course. I mostly oversaw the construction and equipping of my research lab, wrote applications for research grants, wrote articles for publication based on my PhD research, and began mentoring three first-year doctoral students.

At the start of my second year, I arrived fifteen minutes early for the first lecture of my very own course for upper-level undergraduates. As I was relatively new and unknown on campus, I expected only a small student turnout. The room contained more than fifty seats; maybe just the front few rows would fill up.

Before any students arrived, I began chalking on the blackboard an elaborate, multicolored sketch illustrating how an animal's eyes detect an approaching enemy, how its brain processes the received visual information, and how the brain's calculations lead it to respond with either fight or flight. My sketch would provide an overview of the brain's functioning, which we would then explore more deeply throughout the semester.

As I completed my drawing, students began filtering into the room behind me, chatting, laughing, taking their seats. I imagined that some thought I was a teaching assistant and that the professor, older for sure, would show up on the hour. They sounded like a larger audience than I had anticipated, but focusing on my sketch, I didn't yet turn around. Finally, I did and, to my surprise, nearly every seat was filled.

I stepped up to the podium, forced a smile, shuffled my lecture notes, looked up at the class, reshuffled. The students hushed, notebooks open, pens in hand, eyes on me.

"Hi, I'm Jeff Camhi. Welcome to The Brain and Animal Behavior."

I had my next sentence planned, but when I opened my mouth, nothing came out.

I tried again.

Nothing.

I inhaled deeply and tried to force out words as I exhaled. But the only words in my head were my father's voice saying, "Shame on you, shame on you ..."

Seconds ticked by.

Students shared glances.

They spoke in hushed tones.

After what seemed like forever, I managed to blurt out, "Sorry, I'm not feeling well enough to give this lecture," and I dropped into a vacant seat in the front row, staring at my fight-or-flight drawing on the blackboard.

The students murmured, jostled, and began shuffling out of the room. Some approached me with kind words: "Feel better," or "Can I help?"

"No, thanks. Must be my thyroid acting up again. I just need to go home and rest." Thyroid? Rest? Would anyone believe that?

I managed to drive home, where Jane flashed me an anxious look. I recounted what had happened. "Don't worry, we'll get to the bottom of this," she declared.

But I sensed it must be a brain tumor. How would we "get to the bottom" of *that*?

The next morning, she drove me to the doctor. I hadn't finished describing to him what had happened when he uttered, "A clear case of acute anxiety neurosis."

He said I should see a psychiatrist and gave us a recommendation.

* * *

Dr. Feinstein, who introduced himself as Howard, sat opposite me, lanky and relaxed in a brown turtleneck, tan corduroys, and sandals. He spent a lot of time saying little, mostly fingering his long beard, black with a few gray strands.

"What will your treatment be?" My voice wobbled as I imagined all sorts of invasive methods.

"We'll just talk. Mostly you'll talk. About yourself. I'll listen, and once in a while I'll ask a question."

I couldn't have known then that I would talk and he would listen for the next three years. Never in my life had I talked so much. Never had anyone listened so much. Howard would often respond to something I said by asking, "How did that make you feel?" Rarely had anyone asked me that.

During that first year, I saw Howard privately twice a week and met with one of his therapy groups twice a week. Soon Jane and I also joined his married couples' group, also meeting twice a week. Therapy took over my life, while Jane took over almost everything else in our lives, almost always ungrudgingly.

For the first half year, I didn't go back to work at all. Remarkably, the university kept my paychecks coming. "We know you have a great future here," my department head told me, "so whenever you're ready—not before—come on back." I would forever feel grateful for his and Cornell's support. I returned to work after six months, gradually gaining a measure of confidence.

A year after my first attempt to teach my own course, I stood once again at that same podium, a copy of the same fight-or-flight drawing sketched on the board behind me. This time, though still in therapy, quite confidently I led the students through the drawing and through the whole course. Not only did I enjoy the teaching, but I sensed that the students did too.

During my second year in therapy, I saw Howard less frequently and still less in the third year. I gradually came to feel confident and comfortable with myself and with others. From then on, I would regard my three years of therapy as the foundation of my adult life.

* * *

Toward the end of my therapy, Jane suggested we buy a house. She had figured out that with our meager savings, loans from family, and a mortgage, we could just about manage it. A realtor showed us an aging, white clapboard farmhouse on eleven hillside acres with a spring-fed swimming pond and a valley view of pastures and woods. The price seemed manageable. I imagined all that natural beauty embracing us every day. Summers, we would swim in the pond, cook and eat dinner on the terrace, watch the sun set beyond the valley. Winters, we would ski cross-country through our own woods and fields. Even before we signed, Jane was plotting where to plant her vegetable garden, and I had noted where I could erect a backboard and hoop.

The first night in our house, with five-year-old Jeremy asleep in his new upstairs bedroom, I dug a radio out of a box on our living room floor, tuned in to a popular music station, and held Jane in a dance position. They were playing the score of *My Fair Lady*—music that I often played on the piano—and, laughing, I steered us around the jumble of furniture and unopened cartons.

"You're quite the stepper," she complimented.

"Don't forget, my fair lady, those dance lessons I had in my teens."

"Weren't those lessons to get you ready for that girlfriend you took to your senior prom?"

"Actually, I think they were getting me ready for this very moment." I planted a kiss on her lips. I had my woman in my arms, we had our own house, our son was asleep upstairs, and both my university work and Jane's PhD were going well.

I could have danced all night.

* * *

Days later, my mood plummeted. I'd made some quick calculations and realized that, with my ongoing payments to Howard on top of our mortgage and loan payments, we weren't going to make ends meet.

"Next week will be my last therapy session," I told Jane, explaining my calculations.

"No, it won't," she countered. She'd made some calculations of her own and announced that I would continue with Howard for as long as I needed, as long as I wanted. She'd made a change.

"A change?"

Although her doctoral thesis was more than half finished, she was putting it on hold. She'd had a job interview.

"A job?"

Stunned, I wrapped my arms around her. "But your research, it's what you love."

She looked at me, "No, my dear, what I love is you."

She had seen an ad for the administrative director of Cornell's Center for International Studies. She'd phoned to inquire, gone for an interview, and walked out with the job.

Jane loved that job and held it for some time. After I had finished my sessions with Howard, she went back to her doctoral research, although she made a radical change in her thesis subject from medieval history to modern American feminist history, reflecting her growing commitment to the feminist movement.

At that time, Jane was also hired for a year as a part-time lecturer in history at what was then called Cortland State Teachers College. Like me at Cornell, Jane's Cortland job was the first time she had ever taught a course. To my surprise, the night before every lecture she would panic, staying up all hours, working on the lecture's flow. What's the main point? What's an example of it? What resulted from it? What's the next point? Sometimes, still with uncertainties, she would give up, go to sleep for a few hours, and then in the morning class, just wing it. She was smart enough for that, and most often it worked.

I couldn't figure why it was so difficult for her to organize a lecture. It reminded me of some earlier difficulties she had told me about. How, as a Barnard undergraduate, when assigned to write an essay, she was often stumped about how to organize the subject's various points. Her father had helped her with those assignments. She never told me how he helped her, and whether each finished product was really her work or his.

| 4 |

East

After Jane's work, first at Cornell's Center for International Studies and then teaching at Cortland, she wanted to get involved in something "a little more Jewish," as she put it. She applied for a job as director of the Hillel Jewish students' program at nearby Ithaca College. Although she'd taken some courses on Jewish history at Barnard and Berkeley, she'd never engaged in intensive Jewish study. Yet, she got the job.

Her job included organizing Shabbat (sabbath) services on Friday evenings in the college's lovely chapel, which drew a substantial group of students as well as Jeremy and me. After each Friday's service, the three of us drove home, Jane lit Shabbat candles and chanted the traditional blessing over wine, after which we three shared a relaxing Friday night meal. Recognizing Shabbat as a special occasion was new to me. I felt myself being drawn gently, comfortably into a meaningful connection with Judaism, unlike anything I'd experienced before.

* * *

Beginning at age six, I spent nine summers, with Al at a Jewish camp in the Berkshire hills of Massachusetts. Everyone at camp was Jewish, but there was nothing else Jewish about the place—little talk of religion or of Israel.

In eleventh grade, my high school elected me as its representative to the American Field Service foreign exchange program. I was sent to Germany, where I lived for the summer with a German family in a small village near Dusseldorf. During the several months before going, I studied German by means of language-lesson long-play records and achieved a basic conversational level. There were several subjects about which not a word was spoken that summer of 1957: Nazis, the Holocaust, the war, Israel, my being Jewish.

As an undergraduate at Tufts, I joined a Jewish fraternity. It was summer camp all over again: nearly everyone was Jewish, but in those four years, I recall almost no talk of Judaism, no religious traditions, and no mention of Israel.

In sum, while growing up, I didn't feel Judaism or Israel as particularly relevant to my life. However, Jane and her Shabbat services, candle lighting at home, and Friday night dinners were beginning to kindle my interest.

* * *

After fourteen years at Cornell and promotion to tenured full professor, it was time for my second yearlong sabbatical leave. We had spent my first sabbatical at Oxford University, UK, and I thought that this next one could be at Cambridge, UK. I would spend the year trying to complete the textbook I'd been writing on animal behavior and neurobiology.

Jane had an idea different from the UK, however: Jerusalem. Wanting to engage in some in-depth Jewish study, she could think of no better place. Not only would she enhance her professional skills as Hillel director, but also she would feel personally fulfilled. I had met some excellent neurobiology scholars from the Hebrew University of Jerusalem at international conferences, and I agreed that Israel would be a fascinating place to visit.

Jane wondered how to interest fifteen-year-old Jeremy in the idea. Aware of his love of world history and cultures, she presented the idea thus: "You'll be walking where Abraham walked, where King David ruled, and where, not long ago, the Jewish people recreated itself." She was talking his language.

I made inquiries at the Hebrew University and received an invitation to spend the year in their neurobiology department. So, at the start of summer vacation, we packed our bags and left for a year's adventure.

* * *

Jane enrolled in Pardes, an egalitarian yeshiva whose open-minded educational environment suited her well. Her study program extended from early morning to evening, and Jane thrived on it.

Jeremy was enrolled in high school and quickly learned Hebrew. By the end of the year, he had made some close friends and even wished he could stay in Israel to finish high school.

I almost completed my textbook. But for

me, the year's experiences were much broader than my writing. I had come to know people whose life experiences were very different from mine—so many who had suffered the loss of a family member or close friend in the Holocaust, or in a war or terrorist attack. Remarkably, in spite of their life-long grief, many had pushed themselves to return to a full life and contribute to building the state. Israel seemed a nation resting on springs—the harder it was pushed down, the more strongly it bounced back up.

Something else moved me deeply that year. Something that occurred at sunset each Friday when the muted tone of sirens rang out briefly across the land declaring not an emergency but the onset of Shabbat—not Shabbat as we had known it in Ithaca but twenty-four hours of sublime, collective, restful observance.

We observed Shabbat that year at home with a Friday night dinner, often inviting guests, including Jane's Pardes friends. We took on some traditional observances that were new to me. Jane set our Shabbat dinner table beautifully, with the candles, two braided challah breads under a traditional cloth cover, a bottle of good red wine, and a special kiddush cup for the blessing over wine. We would begin by singing the traditional introductory song in Hebrew. As I didn't know the words, I just hummed along. Then we all stood as I filled the kiddush cup, lifted it, and recited in halting Hebrew the blessing that Jane had taught me, following which Jane said the blessing over the bread, and the meal began.

Toward the end of the year, Jane and I began talking about what it would be like when we returned to the States after our intense and fulfilling experience in Israel. I mentioned that I would like to return to Jerusalem now and then for brief visits. "How brief?" Jane asked. I had no answer.

With our departure date back to the States approaching, the president of the Hebrew University invited me to his office and, to my great surprise, offered me a full professorship. Unbeknownst to me, some of the scientists with whom I'd spent the year had made a case on my behalf.

When I told Jane about the offer, she threw her arms around me excitedly. Then, calming down a little, she asked, "What did you tell him?"

"I thanked him very much and told him I would think about it."

"You told him *what?*"

* * *

Returning to Ithaca, we settled back effortlessly into our house on the hill and resumed our former lives. Jane tended to both her vegetable garden and her Hillel students. Jeremy entered his last year of high school, cycled impressive distances, and, come winter, split a great many logs for our woodstove. I returned to directing the research in my lab and teaching my courses.

All was as it had been. All was good.

But not entirely.

I missed the way that Shabbat could switch an entire nation into a state of serenity.

I missed being among people to whom I felt connected by shared history and culture.

Mostly, though, I missed being in a place where being Jewish mattered.

Yet how could I leave Cornell, where things were going so smoothly? Leave Cornell, which had been there for me earlier in my time of need?

I knew that Jane was feeling unsettled. I half expected her to slather cream cheese on a square saltine cracker and, once again, gouge a route from the USA to Jerusalem.

Late one afternoon in my office, in the midst of typing a research paper, I opened my appointment book. Listed for the coming week were a department meeting, committee meetings, a visiting scientist to greet, course lectures to present, seminars to attend, grant applications to submit, research articles to write, and the election of a new departmental chair—all in all, a fairly typical week.

I was forty-one years old.

The second half of my life lay before me.

Where did I want to plant my feet?

* * *

The sun had already set by the time I arrived home, uncharacteristically late, for dinner. Jane met me at the door, head tilted, brow furrowed. "Where have you been?"

"Someplace."

"Where?"

"Pretty far away."

She waited for an explanation.

"Somewhere over there," I said, pointing my finger. "You know, east."

She looked blank.

Then, ever so slowly, her head straightened,

her hands reached toward me, and her lips widened into a broad smile. *"East?"*

I nodded, taking her hands in mine.

I flashed back to that first time I met her in the hallway outside my apartment at Harvard. Ever since she climbed through my window and got me to exercise at 6:00 a.m., supported me through my crisis at Cornell, got us to buy our house, to spend a year in Jerusalem, and in so many other ways Jane had given our lives direction. It was thanks to her that we were now directing our shared gaze to the east, where we planned to spend the rest of our lives.

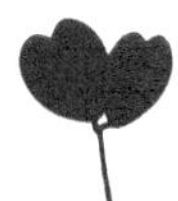

| 5 |

Parents Again?

Jane was hired as an administrator at Pardes, where she had studied during our sabbatical year. There, among other projects, she also created a magazine about people all over Israel who helped other people. Jeremy spent a year working in agriculture and studying Judaism, then joined the Israel Defense Forces for his three years' mandatory military service. Meanwhile, we bought, renovated, and moved into a house in downtown Jerusalem.

A little over a year after we moved in, Jane began volunteering one day a week in a hospital for disabled infants and children. One day, she asked me to come to the hospital to meet a certain seven-month-old boy. He was born with spina bifida, causing both permanent paralysis and a total lack of sensation from his lower abdomen to his toes. His parents had abandoned him at birth and neither they nor any of their family or friends came to visit him. The hospital was his home, the nurses his family.

"I'm really busy these days, dear" was my reply.

"Yes, I know, but maybe just a brief visit," she replied.

The following week she asked me again. And again a third week.

"Okay, a brief visit," I ultimately replied.

"Great. Wait till you see his ear-to-ear smile, his big, bright, brown eyes. Till you feel his tight hug when you hold him—to me it feels electric."

I hadn't thought about actually holding him. It had been a long time since I'd held a baby.

Arriving at the hospital, I spotted Jane at the far end of a corridor, a baby in her arms. I walked in their direction, but slowly, peeking into side rooms along the way, scanning a bulletin board, reading a few posted notices.

"We're over here, Jeff. Keep coming. You can do it." When I arrived, "Jeff, meet Alon."

She was right about his big smile, his bright eyes. She surprised me by placing him in my arms. He hugged me tightly around my neck, and I felt that electricity she'd talked about. I jiggled him and he smiled; I did it again and he laughed. I carried him into a playroom, where we both got down, bellies on floor, and rolled a rubber ball back and forth with much giggling. Lying there with him reminded me of playing Walnut on the floor with Jeremy. For Alon, though, belly-down was the only option. Jane had explained to me that he lacked the lower back support needed for sitting up.

Jane and I visited Alon a few more times in the following weeks. Then we started going twice a week, spending a few hours with him each time.

One day, we peeked into Alon's room, where he lay belly-down in his crib, his face turned away from us. As we approached, I whispered his name. He turned his head toward us. An incipient smile quickly turned to a pout. Then to tears. And then to screams.

What had happened? Had I misunderstood his feelings about us? Was he not enjoying our visits? Did he want us to leave?

Then it dawned on me. Alon seemed to be screaming, in the only language he knew, "Where the hell have you been?"

I picked him up.

Our faces touched.

His tears mixed with mine.

When we left the hospital that day and got into the car, I paused before inserting the ignition key. I turned to Jane and announced, "Our visits here are a problem."

She stared at me, slack-jawed, her hands raised with palms toward me as if defending herself from my words.

"No, I don't mean we should stop. The opposite. Our visits must be confusing him. He doesn't know who he belongs to, the nurses or us. I think he should be ours, full time, at home."

Reaching out to me, Jane stroked my cheeks, pulled me toward her, and planted her soft, warm lips on my forehead. She didn't say a word.

We both knew. Twenty years after Jeremy's birth, once again we were about to become parents.

* * *

Adoption of an abandoned child was a complex process, but we were guided each step of the way by remarkable social workers at both the hospital and Israel's Child Welfare Service. The biggest problem was that Alon's biological parents refused not only to take him home but also to release him for adoption or even for fostering. The Child Welfare Service took the biological parents to court, where the judge offered them two options: either take Alon home and raise him as their son or permit us to do so. They chose the latter option. Thus, just before his first birthday, Alon became our foster child and moved out of the hospital into our home. About a year later, he became our legally adopted child.

In Hebrew, Alon means oak tree, and indeed, Jane and I sensed his inner oak-like strength. Before he'd left the hospital, Alon was fitted with a firm body brace that allowed him to sit up straight and strong, just like an oak. Jane suggested that we give Alon a middle name, and she suggested Moshe (Hebrew for Moses) to signify our plucking him out of the hospital, just as Moses was plucked out of the River Nile. Our new son was thus named Alon Moshe Camhi.

* * *

Alon soon learned to use a wheelchair and to scoot around the house. When he turned three, we took him to the Peto Institute in Budapest, which taught disabled children to use those parts of the body that work to compensate for those parts that don't. Our first day there, they fitted him with a brace on each leg, gave him a low chair so he could hold on to its back, and he then stood for the first time in his life. A few days later they replaced the chair with two tripod-based walking sticks. They then placed a volleyball on the floor in front of him and taught him to lean onto his left leg and swing the right side of his torso forward, which caused his right leg to kick the ball. Next, the same for his left leg. A little later, using those same torso movements, they taught him to take a forward step with his right leg, then his left, and then his right again. Within an hour, Jane and I watched through teary eyes as Alon, fully paralyzed from abdomen to toes, walk across the room using his tripod sticks.

We made five trips to the Peto Institute, each six weeks long. Jane and I split our time there, overlapping for a few days in the middle to share in Alon's progress and to have a brief holiday together. During these trips, Alon's walking ability improved, and he even learned to go up and down stairs. His walking nevertheless remained slow and laborious, suitable only for indoors.

* * *

Despite Alon's many special needs while growing up, his ear-to-ear smile persisted. He could also crack a good joke and set a roomful of people laughing or respond to something said with a remarkably sensitive reply.

We all learned to cope with his modest learning disability, which required an assistant to help him through high school. Following his graduation, he tried to enlist in the army—there were many office jobs he could have fulfilled—but the army didn't care to engage a recruit high in spirit but low in physical capacity. He enrolled in college to study law but decided after a year that it was not for him.

Jane and I tried hard to cope with Alon's many surgeries—twenty-two by the age of twenty-five, several minor, a few major. Many of these surgeries concerned Alon's hydrocephalus, which often accompanies spina bifida. With hydrocephalus, the natural flow of fluid from the cavities deep in the brain and through the spinal cord is partially blocked, putting pressure on the brain tissue. The treatment for this was to install permanently a very thin tube—a shunt— to drain off some of the fluid from the brain's cavities. That treatment worked well, but sometimes the shunt would clog and Alon would suffer intense pain caused by the swelling of his brain's cavities. If not treated swiftly, the ever-increasing pressure on his brain tissue could have been fatal.

It was difficult enough for Jane and me to care for the broad range of Alon's special needs, but our greatest concern was always the shunt and his brain.

* * *

When Alon turned twenty-two, he decided to move into his own apartment nearby. We engaged a full-time live-in helper, Priyantha, from Sri Lanka, who was to remain his long-time caregiver.

About then, Alon began volunteering at a nonprofit organization that assists the elderly and the disabled. There he became a consultant in their implement-lending department. He would meet usually with disabled clients and explain which item was suitable for their needs and how to use it. Alon thrived and continued there for a decade. He loved his supervisors, and they clearly loved him.

I asked Alon one day how he liked his volunteering, and he answered, "It's what I like most in life, helping people in need."

| 6 |

Presents

Throughout our marriage, I marked each of Jane's birthdays with a present and sometimes a party. But when she turned sixty-five, that changed.

"Jeff, don't give me any more birthday presents," she instructed, several weeks before the date. Had she not liked the sweaters, blouses, and scarves that I'd picked out over the years? "And don't make me any more birthday parties," she added. Had I uncorked the wrong wine? Sliced the wrong cake? Invited the wrong people?

Now I had to find some other way to celebrate.

Close to midnight on the eve of her birthday, I got into bed first and slipped something under her pillow. I couldn't hide a little smile as she slid under the covers.

"Have you got some proposition on your mind ...?" she began.

"No, not that," I assured her. "The occasional *preposition*, perhaps." Oops, did that give it away?

She settled herself under the covers, and I waited for her to lift and plump up her pillow—her usual bedtime procedure. But instead she got out of bed and opened a window.

"Jane, it's late November. Do you want us to freeze?"

This was nothing new. She always liked it cold, "more healthy." I liked it warm, "more comfy." That night, as usual, healthy trumped comfy.

Settling back under the covers, she lay flat on her back. I lifted my pillow, giving it an exaggerated plumping, but she didn't take the hint. Rather, she tossed me a goodnight kiss in the air.

"I heard that kiss," I affirmed, "but it sailed straight up to the ceiling and never drifted down to me."

"Oh, okay," she said, and as she turned my way for direct delivery, her elbow slipped under her pillow. "What's this?" She switched on her bedside lamp and smiled at the green envelope with my drawing of a red heart pierced by an arrow. She opened it, pulled out the enclosed page, and recited the typed lines:

A wise man told us someplace far,
"Love each other for what you are,
Forgive each other for what you 'ain't'";
With his advice, I've no complaint.

For I've got you and you've got me,
And so together we've got we.
And I'll be here with you, my love,
Until we head for heav'n above.

And so with you I'll always walk,
Whether we're quiet, whether we talk,
Whether we're smart or whether we're not,
'Cause with you, all I need, I've got.

So hold my hand and I'll hold yours,
For love spills out from all my pores.

Jane wiped the tears from her eyes. "That's so beautiful," she whispered, and we held each other tight.

On each successive birthday, I was to give her no present, no party.

Just a poem.

* * *

On the morning of her birthday, Jane was humming as she busied herself around in the kitchen. That was strange; Jane was not a hummer. But she danced over to me and hummed in my ear the Rodgers and Hammerstein tune "Oh, What a Beautiful Mornin'," the perfect AM song for her birthday, I thought, and we sang together the line about the corn growing high, clear up to the sky. We grabbed hands, and she repeated that line, but with one minor change, namely that it was *we* who were climbin' clear up to the sky.

I didn't get it.

She just kept smiling as we prepared breakfast.

"Is there something you want to tell me?" I asked.

"Oh, just a little something. Maybe later."

But she couldn't wait.

"You and I are going trekking up Annapurna."

"Excuse me?"

"Mount Annapurna. It's in the Himalayas."

"Yes, I know what it is. And where."

I felt her throbbing excitement. Mountains

were Jane. Climbing the Adirondacks in her youth, guiding teenage summer campers up New Hampshire's White Mountains during her college years, strolling with me—at the easy pace I could manage—on summer vacations in the Adirondacks, the Rockies, the Alps. But now, on the morning of her sixty-fifth birthday, she was laying claim to the most challenging ascent of her life.

"You're going to love this trip," she proclaimed.

Me climbing Annapurna? I knew that wasn't going to happen. But how could I crush her dream? Especially after I'd written her a poem that claimed, "And so with you I'll always walk!"

"Jane, I need to tell you something," I uttered.

That was all she needed to hear. Her head slumped. Her shoulders drooped. Her chest deflated. She turned away, picked up a dishtowel, and started wiping dishes that had already lain overnight on the drain board. More than once she wiped her face.

I came up behind and put my arms around her. But she pulled away, walked around me and into the living room, sat on the couch, and picked up the morning's *Jerusalem Post*.

How could I spoil the film she had created in her mind with me cast as her costar?

But I knew I couldn't do it.

I walked into the living room and sat beside her on the couch.

She positioned the fully open *Post* between us.

At first, I said nothing. Then I had a brainwave. I paused, thought about it, and thought again.

"Jane, you wouldn't want me slowing you down. You need someone who can go at your pace or even push you beyond yourself. Someone younger. A natural trekker."

She lowered the *Post* just a bit, then raised it again.

"I've got it," I proclaimed. "You need Naomi!"

Slowly, inch by inch, the *Post* slid downward. I glimpsed her hair, then her forehead, and her eyes squinting as though trying to picture Naomi with her, there on Annapurna.

Her eyes widened. "Naomi," she murmured.

A professional fitness coach, twenty years Jane's junior, Naomi loved mountain climbing. We had come to know her well, years before, when she lived alone in our small basement apartment and served as Alon's helper. Jane had stayed close to her since then.

Single and without children, on receiving Jane's invitation, it took Naomi less than a day to juggle her plans and say yes to the expedition.

Beginning the next day, Jane engaged in a daily training regimen—climbing the steep hills from our house into town, then around Jerusalem's Old City, and back. Once a week, she took a long, ambitious walk in the Judean Hills with her friend Laura, also an avid hiker. This regimen lasted several months.

"What about possible dangers in the Himalayas?" I asked Jane one evening. "You know, narrow cliffside trails with steep drop-offs, snowstorms, avalanches, little stuff like that?"

She just shrugged.

Some weeks later, Jane flew off with Naomi. Narrow cliffside trails, snowstorms, and the rest were on my mind all the time she was gone.

Five weeks later she returned, proclaiming, "It was the high point of my life. And not just in an altitudinal sense." She brought home a photo that captured her spirit of adventure and achievement. Standing proud, high on an Annapurna ledge, she was gazing outward toward distant snow-covered peaks, squinting against the bright sunshine. I framed that photo and placed it on my baby grand piano. Every time I sat at the keyboard, I caught sight of her, climbin' clear up to the sky.

* * *

"What's that you're so glued to?" I asked Jane one afternoon as she sprawled on the living room couch, a book in one hand, a pen in the other. She didn't answer.

I asked again.

"It's about death," she replied.

I looked at the title on the cover: *The Tibetan Book of Living and Dying*.

"When I die," she said, "lay my body on a mountaintop. Leave it there for the birds to peck at."

Just like Jane, I thought, wanting to end on a peak. But why was she suddenly so concerned with her end? Besides, given that I didn't think I couldn't walk with her up Annapurna, how on earth was I going to lug her body up a mountain? I was pretty sure she didn't mean it literally, though, probably just a thought triggered by her increasing turn toward Buddhism.

Recalling the Buddhist justice of the peace who had married us, I asked her, if she died but I couldn't heft her up a mountain, would she then "forgive me for what I ain't?"

"Oh, that was Chinese Buddhism," she laughed. "This is Tibetan."

I wasn't aware of the fine distinctions. In fact, I knew very little about Buddhism.

Jane, though, was becoming both involved and knowledgeable. She joined a Buddhist study and meditation group, a *sangha*, that met once a week, and she started attending Buddhist retreats. When the Dalai Lama and other illustrious Buddhist leaders lectured in Israel, she took me to hear them. I found them interesting. Jane found them life-changing. Soon she was referring to herself as a "Jew-Bu" and explained that there was no real conflict; you could be both, particularly since Buddhism has no supreme being to conflict with the Jewish God—a God I wasn't quite sure in which she believed.

Jane never came right out and said whether or not she believed in God, or whether she shared my disbelief. Strange, because we generally talked freely about any subject. Her God reticence left me wondering whether there might be other things she wasn't telling me.

* * *

Nearly five years after Jane told me not to give her any more birthday presents, she sent this email to twelve of her closest woman friends:

Thursday, November 23 is coming soon—my 70th birthday. I invite you all, who are very dear to me, to a gathering at my home for an evening salon rather than a party. This way I won't have to keep you entertained and can just be in the moment. I suggest that the conversation include issues of life and death, significant turning points, definitive moments, our sense of self and where it comes from, our satisfactions and disappointments (what we would do differently), how we feel about aging, our spiritual proclivities, insights, and struggles. I hope the appended readings—essays, short fiction pieces, and poems—will help give our discussion direction. Jane was not one for small talk.

The gathering was so successful that it became a regular monthly event for the next five years, each month hosted by a different member. As the unofficial chair, Jane sought a name for the group. She tried out some options on me: "To Age and to Sage," for instance. I was not enthusiastic. Too cumbersome. She changed it to "Aging and Saging." Tighter, I thought; it could work. Ultimately, she abbreviated it to "A&S."

A fine wine and a great meal contributed by all the participants added to the success of each A&S gathering. So too, the decision that any male partner of the hosting A&S member would be out of the house for the evening.

Like many of Jane's undertakings, the creation of A&S had a significant effect on me. It served as a model for a parallel men's group that I organized with a friend, which would also meet monthly. We thought carefully about who to invite into the group: men who would be interested in and capable of openly sharing their intimate thoughts and feelings; men who would listen closely to one another and not interrupt; men who would not talk during our sessions about the stock market, sports, politics, or their work. Men who, we realized, might be hard to find.

Ultimately, we invited five men to join, ranging in age from age fifty-five to eighty, and we met monthly, ultimately for eight years. We never lacked for subjects to discuss.

PART II

DESCENT

Kyoto

"You cook dinner tonight, okay?" Jane asked. "I'm just so ... I don't know ..."

"Wiped out from our long flight? Me too. But sure, I can throw some veggies into a wok."

It was early June 2009. Jane and I had just arrived at the apartment we had rented for a month in Kyoto, Japan, after two wonderful weeks in Hawaii. We were celebrating my retirement from the Hebrew University at the prescribed age of sixty-eight. This trip was to mark the boundary between the research and teaching life I was leaving behind and some exciting activities that lay ahead. One of those, in fact, was located at the university, so I would still be going there on a semiregular basis.

For our first Kyoto dinner, I chopped and mixed the strange foods we'd just bought in a local outdoor market: several exotically shaped vegetables, moist gray cubes that we believed to be fish, little round nuts, a sweet tasting orange goo, and a red liquid that made my eyes water the moment I opened the bottle. I spooned and dribbled them all into a hot, oiled wok.

Over the sizzling sounds, I heard Jane flipping TV channels in the living room. Nothing in English. Then she held one channel for a few minutes.

"What are you watching?" I called out.

"Sumo wrestling."

"Yeah? Those half-naked fat fellas turn you on?"

No answer. But she popped into the kitchen, kissed my cheek, and whispered, "Nope, only you."

She shook her head, sniffing the aromas swirling up and out of the wok.

"How do you know what to do with all this stuff?"

I put her question down to this being her first time in Japan, whereas I had twice attended conferences in Tokyo and had at least seen and sampled various local foods. I whooshed the mixture around, splashed in some soy sauce, and served us our first Kyoto dinner.

* * *

The next morning, we headed out to a well-known Buddhist temple nearby. Three young priests wrapped in orange robes walked barefoot on a sea of white gravel, raking it into a wavy pattern of parallel furrows.

"I've read that they do this every morning," Jane whispered, "and each day they create a different design."

As we rounded a corner, she let out a deep sigh: "Look at this, Jeff, have you ever seen such a perfect garden?" A ground cover of mosses surrounded three large, craggy rocks, a spring-fed pool with large, multicolored koi fish, a stunted Japanese maple tree, and a path of beautiful, irregularly shaped stones inviting us through lush, leafy ferns and pointed horsetails.

"If only my sangha could meet here," she ruminated, "we'd probably never leave. I'm so glad we chose Kyoto. I feel at peace here."

Back in the apartment, jet lag hit us, and we lay down for a nap. When I awoke, Jane was sitting up in bed, beads of perspiration studding her forehead. Despite the air conditioner's cooling blast, she was waving her blouse out away from her chest for ventilation.

"What's wrong? Are you sick?"

"Last night's dinner." She turned to me, then jerked her head away, then turned back to me.

"Really? Was something spoiled?" I berated myself for shopping at that open market. "Maybe it was that cubed fish-like stuff."

"No. Not that. It's ... well, it's ..."

"What?"

"Oh, piss. It's that I couldn't have cooked it myself."

"You were tired, dear, I knew that. Of course you could. It's the easiest thing. You just throw stuff into the wok, stir, and fry. That's why they call it stir-fry."

"Don't joke! Sometimes ..." She opened another button of her blouse. "Sometimes I'm not sure what to put in when." This from the woman who had cooked most of our meals for nearly fifty years.

"What and when? That's easy." I reached for the pen and pad on my bedside table. Across the top, I scrawled, "STIR-FRY," and then, "1) Oil." It was like writing a lab protocol for one of my research students.

"For God's sake, don't!" she protested. "You just do the cooking while we're here, and I'll clean up afterward, okay? I'm sorry."

This being our vacation, I decided yes to cook, no to complain. Whatever the problem, I'd wait for it to subside or for Jane to bring it up again. Meanwhile, I became chef for a month.

* * *

Since our fridge was only slightly larger than a shoebox, we continued making almost daily trips to the market. We would step out of our apartment building and head along our narrow side street lined with private row houses, each painted a different pastel color. Small, manicured front gardens, rich in mosses, ferns, and horsetails, some even incorporating tiny patches of raked white or gray gravel, recalled the temple gardens. These lovely homes and gardens lent a measure of beauty, perhaps even spirituality, to the onset of each excursion from our apartment.

We soon approached a T-junction onto a busy commercial boulevard with bumper-to-bumper traffic, engine exhaust, and the bustle of people walking in and out of the many small shops. Turning right took us to our landmark Buddhist temple, left led to the market.

On our third or fourth shopping expedition, Jane stopped short at the T-junction and looked left and right and left again. "Which way?" she asked.

"We're going to the market."

"I know. Which way?"

"Jane, you know this junction."

"Don't 'Jane' me! Which way, dammit?"

I sighed. "Left, just like yesterday and the day before that and the day—"

"Okay, okay, don't get pissy about it," she demurred, looking left and right several more times.

What was going on? I took her hand and led her into the shade of a nearby kiosk. "Dear, we haven't stayed for any length of time in a new place since moving to Israel, and that was over twenty-five years ago. Of course everything is unfamiliar here. When we're back in Jerusalem, you'll see, things will click right back to normal."

I was concerned, though, and I decided to keep an eye out for any other signs of confusion. If they were to occur, I would jot down the elapsed time from this Kyoto T-junction moment to each additional occurrence of Jane's confusion.

* * *

I wondered whether we should go ahead with the following day's plan. If Jane was having some sort of problem, Hiroshima was perhaps the last place she should visit. I searched my memory about our recent stay in Hawaii when we had spent a somber day visiting Pearl Harbor. Were there any hints from that visit?

What had touched both of us most deeply there was the memorial to the battleship USS *Arizona*. We gathered with other visitors on a floating gallery built right over the sunken ship that had gone down with more than one thousand sailors. As if sending messages up from the deep, bubbles of oil from within the hull were still rising to the surface after all those years.

I searched my memory for any signs that may have bubbled up from deep within Jane during our day at Pearl Harbor. As I recalled none, I sensed that we could go ahead with our plan for Hiroshima.

We boarded the famous bullet train, and remarkably soon, we disembarked and took a bus that dropped us a short walk from the Peace Memorial Park. It was a fine sunny day, and the city looked lovely—that is, until we arrived at the Genbaku Dome building, bombed-out and lying there still in ruins. The centerpiece of

Hiroshima's Memorial Park, this building commemorated the deaths of perhaps one hundred thousand people from that instantaneous blast.

An elderly woman in a green floral kimono called out a soft hello from a bench and asked in heavily accented English whether we would like an explanation. She clarified that she was not a tour guide and would request no payment. We sat down beside her.

She had been just four when the bomb was dropped, she said, on the morning of August 6, 1945. That meant she was my age. She had been staying at her grandparents' house some distance from the city, but her parents had been at home in downtown Hiroshima and were killed instantly. Her grandparents raised her from then on. Jane reached out and touched her hand.

"I have health problem from that day. Weakness. Trouble to walk."

Jane squeezed her hand.

"We must each look inward to find our deep strength," the woman said.

"Yes," Jane replied.

I felt as though I were sitting in on one of Jane's A&S meetings.

"Also we must look outward and share our love," the woman continued.

"Yes, yes," Jane whispered. The conversation went on for some twenty minutes, and when we all stood up, Jane and the woman hugged. Jane dabbed her eyes as we walked across the park to the Peace Memorial Museum.

Of all the museum's exhibits, one small object particularly affected us both. A wall-mounted clock, badly damaged, its hands stuck at the time 8:15 pointed to the decisive moment of that dreadful morning's explosion. Everything can change in a split second, I realized

Riding home on the bullet train, Jane and I reflected on what we had heard and seen. I also reflected privately on how well Jane had coped with the day's deeply emotional moments, seeming fully herself. If she could endure such painful emotions as we'd experienced that day, what was there for me to worry about?

Back in Kyoto, we took a bus that let us off at the T-junction near our apartment. It was still light out, and the market would still be open. I suggested we walk there and buy food for dinner. Jane agreed.

"Which way?" she asked.

| 8 |

Keys

"Stop! This isn't the way we go!" Jane exclaimed, fumbling in her handbag and pulling out her sunglasses. "You made a wrong turn somewhere."

It was several months since we'd returned home from Kyoto. We were on our way to visit Jeremy, his wife Ariela, and our three grandkids in their home, half an hour from Jerusalem. We had first picked up Alon from his apartment.

"Jane, we usually head to Jeremy's house from our place, not Alon's. That's why it seems different now. Look, there's the Central Bus Station." I pointed a forefinger from my grip on the steering wheel. "Don't you recognize it?"

"You're in the whole wrong part of town, dammit. What are you doing?"

Alon reached his hand over the back of Jane's seat and gently stroked her shoulder.

"It's all right, Mom. This is one of the ways to Jeremy's." Jane calmed down a bit. But in the rearview mirror, I saw Alon's head swaying left and right—a sure sign of his agitation. Watching him, I went through a red light and nearly rammed into a taxi. The driver shouted at me through his open window and zoomed away.

I tried to shake this off. I'd driven plenty over the years and never had an accident. I had never especially enjoyed driving, though; for me, it was just what you have to do to get where you're going.

For Jane, though, a car had always meant adventure. In college she'd read Kerouac's *On the Road* about his escapades crisscrossing the States on backstreets. Then one summer, she did the same with her college roommate in her beat-up Ford. They spent a week on a native American reservation in Arizona and then cruised through sleepy towns in the Deep South singing freedom songs out of open car windows. "Not so smart," I'd commented when Jane first told me this. When we'd lived in Ithaca, Jane thought nothing of driving alone four and a half hours north to see her childhood friends in Saranac Lake or the same distance south to visit her mother in Manhattan. In Israel too, for several years she had driven up and down the country to interview people for the magazine she'd created when she'd worked at Pardes.

Jane belonged in the driver's seat, and when she drove, I imagined Kerouac was riding shotgun.

But lately, she'd been asking me to run errands that she would normally have happily carried out. And when we entered the car to drive any distance, while earlier she would often take the wheel, now she edged into the passenger's seat but said nothing about it.

* * *

Then one day, about a month after our visit to Jeremy's, the phone rang in my university office. "When are you coming home?" Jane's voice quivered.

"Just winding things up here. Maybe an hour or so. Why?"

"Come now!"

I hailed a cab and was there in fifteen minutes.

Jane sat slumped on the couch, wet tissues crumpled in her lap.

I wrapped my arm around her shoulders.

"I was driving someplace. Over there," she said, her voice trembling as she pointed a limp finger this way and that, "and I was in a long, dark tunnel, and it had no end, and the road was a black ribbon, and it was curling up over me, about to crush me, and I couldn't breathe."

She grasped her throat, and her whole body shuddered. I tightened my grip on her shoulders.

"I left the car after the tunnel—I don't remember the name of the street. I got out and there was a taxi and I got in, but I forgot our address and I said, 'Go this way,' you know, I pointed, and I was right and I got home and I called you."

She rocked back and forth, sobbing, as I pulled her toward me.

Later that day, when she remembered the name of the street, I went and retrieved the car.

* * *

"She has to stop driving," Dr. Ban said when I consulted him the next morning. He'd been our family doctor for over twenty years—a short man, late sixties, with sparse graying hair, narrow-rimmed glasses, and a gray mustache hovering over thin, smiling lips. No white coat, no framed medical degrees on his walls, though we knew he'd trained at the best American medical schools and hospitals and was frequently consulted by his colleagues about their most challenging cases.

"She won't stop driving," I asserted. "You know how she loves popping off here and there. Take that away and she'd feel paralyzed."

Taking away Jane's car keys would also make me the designated driver for all family needs, including shopping and other errands. I was already feeling the strain of that growing role, and I wasn't eager for it to increase.

"But she could get confused again and hurt somebody," the doctor continued. "Or herself. Or worse."

That did it. I needed no more convincing.

But how could I tell her?

That night, as we sat together in the living room, an idea popped into my mind—a long shot but worth a try. "Jane," I began, "remember all those hikes you used to take with Laura when you were getting in shape for your Annapurna trek? Each time you came back from a hike, you felt so energized."

"Yeah, so?"

"Well, when Laura went to tour guide school,

I'll bet she learned about many trails all around and through Jerusalem—in fact, all over the country. Why don't you see if she'd like to go for walks with you again? Maybe once or twice a week. I bet she'd love that."

"Where's this going?"

"Well, you know how driving has become kind of a problem for you."

"Stop it! You want me to walk instead of drive? Go away. Leave me alone!"

Next, I wondered whether Dr. Ban could reach her. He agreed to give it a try. But how to get her to his office? I told her that he had a medication that may prevent another frightening incident while she was driving. She didn't seem to catch wind of my little fib.

"Jane, I know how much you care about people," Dr. Ban began.

She turned to face me, peering at him out the corners of her eyes.

He told her he'd read some of the articles she used to write for Pardes about people who help others and he also knew how she herself helped people. Especially Alon, he added.

She turned to him. "So?"

"Well, I know the last thing you would ever want is to hurt someone."

Jane breathed deeply through flared nostrils.

"But from what I can see, you could actually hurt someone if you keep on driving."

She shot out of her chair. "Oh piss ... You're not taking away my car keys! Who the hell ...!" She swung open the office door and bolted down the hall. That was the first time I noticed something strange about her walking. I couldn't tell what exactly, but her steps were just a bit short, a bit irregular. At one point she reached out and balanced herself against the wall. Probably just stressed about the driving, I assumed. She walked right past the lobby, and only when she reached the exit door did she turn around and find her way back to a chair. There she sat, rocking back and forth, glaring in my direction along the hallway and through the open office door.

Dr. Ban turned to me. "Jeff, I know how difficult all this must be for you. So tell me, how are you feeling?"

His question caught me off guard. Our close friends had been asking me about Jane, but few had asked about me, and now I didn't really have an answer. I just looked down at my hands. All I could think to say was, "Fine, actually."

"Okay, but when you're not feeling 'fine actually,' I'm here."

* * *

My further attempts to broach the driving subject with Jane failed miserably. Finally, Alon suggested I tell her that she might end up hurting someone she really cares about, like Dr. Ban himself, if she kept driving.

Leave it to Alon to think of such a personal solution.

The next time Jane and I were sitting together quietly on the couch, I remarked, "Dear, you know if you keep on driving, Dr. Ban could lose his medical license."

She pulled a *Jerusalem Post* from the coffee table, opened it wide, and pretended to be reading. "What do you mean?" she asked.

I told her that it is a doctor's responsibility to remove unsteady drivers from the road. A doctor who doesn't do that can be sued in court and might never be able to practice medicine again. I had no idea whether this was true, but I continued that if she should, by any chance, hit someone on the road, Dr. Ban's career could be over. I added for good measure that we would then lose him as our doctor.

Jane put the newspaper down and sat there quietly. Then she stood up and started walking toward her study. This time I noticed something even stranger about her gait. It was as though she were crossing a stream by stepping on a series of protruding rocks and gauging precisely on which rock to position each step.

I followed her. At the entrance to her study she stopped short, took a deep breath, then turned and approached the study's far wall, where her handbag hung from a hook. With another deep breath, she poked her hand deep inside it and then stood there for some time, perfectly still, her back to me.

My heart was pounding. In my mind, I saw Kerouac nodding goodbye to Jane, opening the passenger door, stepping out, scratching his scruffy beard, shielding his eyes from the desert sun, and trudging off across the burning sand, his image shrinking, then disappearing, never to return.

She turned and stepped slowly toward me.

She reached out and lifted my hand.

Gazing straight into my eyes, she placed her car keys in my palm and closed my fingers over them.

Lowering her eyes, she sidestepped me and returned to the living room.

I heard the rustling of a newspaper.

| 9 |

AD

Over the next few months, there were times when Jane seemed almost her old self, but more and more times when she did not. We hardly ever talked about it; I didn't know what to say, and she seemed just as happy saying nothing.

When Dr. Ban suggested that Jane go for a neuropsychology examination, she put up no resistance. Whatever was afflicting her, it was time we defined it. Even bad news might give us—or at least me—a clearer sense of where we were heading, which might make it easier for us—or at least me—to deal with.

It was about nine months since Kyoto when the neuropsychologist, seated at his tidy desk, invited Jane to sit in the adjacent chair and, turning to his computer, asked for her particulars, with which I helped her, and he typed them in. He then turned toward Jane and, after a few introductory comments, explained, "Here's the first exercise. When I click this button on my stopwatch, you'll have thirty seconds to say as many words starting with F as you can."

"That's too easy," Jane scoffed. Perhaps she wanted a test hard enough to finally reveal her problem and its cause. For her, words were always, as she said, "too easy."

"We'll see," he replied.

Click.

Out wafted the likes of fecundity, felicitous, ferocity, fabrication, foolhardy, the neuropsychologist's eyebrows rising higher with each rapid-fire multisyllable. Jane's last two words almost toppled him: "fornicate, fuck."

I couldn't contain my laughter. Not only was Jane funny, not only was I amused that the neuropsychologist might have landed on the floor, but it was also fun to be reminded of the competent Jane that once was.

For his next test, the neuropsychologist explained that he would tap out some rhythms on his desk and, after each one, she should tap back the same rhythm. She did reasonably well on his first few simple trials, though as his taps grew more syncopated, perhaps expectedly, she became less able to copy their rhythms.

We had come there to find out what specifically was wrong with Jane, and so far, it seemed as though nothing was wrong. Strangely, I was hoping Jane would fail convincingly in at least one exercise so we could come away with a definitive diagnosis, whatever it might be.

Next, he instructed her to draw a clock with its hands showing the time of twenty minutes to six. She drew what looked like the outline of a sweet potato and distributed twelve numbers unevenly around it. She drew the short hour hand pointing to six and the longer minute hand pointing to two. Now we were getting somewhere, I sensed.

After a few more exercises in which Jane partly succeeded, the neuropsychologist turned to his computer, did some calculations, and began typing. He then looked up at Jane. "Your situation appears to be one of age-appropriate cognitive dysfunction. That means that you're just getting a bit older. Nothing to worry about, it happens to us all. See me again in a year." He stood, handed me his typed report, and motioned us to the door.

"As I thought," Jane said when we'd left his office, "just my aging brain."

Yet, there was something in the way she said that, perhaps a lack of self-assurance, almost like a child trying out an idea on a parent while already sensing that the parent would disagree.

But I didn't disagree. I was too busy trying to figure out where to go from there. I had my doubts about this "age-appropriate cognitive dysfunction" idea. And I certainly wasn't going to wait a year for a follow-up. I scheduled a consultation with Dr. Ban for myself alone to ask whom we should see next.

"It can't be just aging," I told him, adding that we're all aging but we don't all get stuck every time we come to a T-junction or sense that we're driving into a tunnel with no end.

Dr. Ban nodded and commented that these tests are not perfect. He had someone else in mind for us to see: a professor of neurology, Dr. Buchman. Unfortunately, though, he was overseas for three months doing research—"on Alzheimer's."

Dr. Ban stared at me as he uttered that "A" word. Maybe he thought I'd be shocked at hearing it. I wasn't. It was the word I'd expected, the one I'd feared, the one that I couldn't shake from my mind. But it was good that he said that word out loud. It was as though his doing so opened a door to a room in which everything seemed broken. Only by looking inside could we determine whether we could make some order of the chaos.

I awaited Dr. Buchman's return.

* * *

A short, chubby man, probably late sixties, stuffed into a wrinkled tan shirt and a brown tweed sport jacket, Dr. Buchman welcomed us with a bearded smile and a gentle voice. He apologized for the book-filled boxes strewn around the floor of his half-empty office. Jane was to be his last patient, he explained; he was retiring from medical practice and would be devoting himself full time to his research. He assured us, however, that we could continue to visit him at his home, as necessary.

Dr. Buchman carried out nearly the same test as the neuropsychologist. But now the thirty-second word test, this time on G words, evoked from Jane mostly monosyllables: "Go, give ... umm, gave, get ... umm, go ..." I was stunned by the decline since her F test only four months previously.

Likewise, in the rhythm test, her tapping on

the desk resembled the random banging of a metal gate in a wind storm. Her clock drawing was right out of Salvador Dali.

While I would have expected Jane to be distressed at how poorly she was doing, she showed no sign of it. She just sat quietly, doing what Dr. Buchman said. Maybe she was concentrating on her answers and had no reserve mental space for disappointment. Or maybe she thought she was responding well.

Dr. Buchman typed up his report, folded it in two, and handed it to me.

As I peeked inside, the words "Probable AD" jumped out at me.

So there it was in black and white—Alzheimer's Dementia. I knew that the word "probable" meant that the only definitive diagnosis of Alzheimer's required a microscopic examination of the brain tissue, carried out postmortem.

I now knew—as well as I would ever know—that Jane had Alzheimer's.

The blessing we had received from the justice of the peace at our first wedding ran through my mind: "Love each other for what you are and forgive each other for what you ain't."

Perhaps most shocking was that Jane would lose most or all of her speech. I remembered that awful moment when I was briefly rendered speechless at the first lecture of my very first course at Cornell.

But Jane, of all people, speechless? Permanently?

* * *

Dr. Ban had advised me not to mention the word *Alzheimer's* to Jane, as that could throw her into a depression. He clarified, though, that this advice raised a moral dilemma for him. Physicians are obligated to give each patient a full and accurate diagnosis so that they can consider available options and decide on a course of action. But he was convinced that Jane was no longer able to consider options, or decide on actions, even if there were relevant actions from which to choose. Dr. Buchman seemed to agree, having used the abbreviation AD in his report. As we left his office, I said to Jane, "It looks like what you've been saying all along, dear, your aging brain."

She stopped, pulled me toward her, and replied, "You mean my brain disorder."

| 10 |

Words Unspoken

My not mentioning Alzheimer's to Jane meshed with the fact that, throughout our marriage, we had rarely talked about death. True, we had occasionally broken that silence, as in her Buddhism-inspired request that I leave her corpse on a mountaintop. Also, in loving moments, she had occasionally implored me: "Please don't go before me. I don't know how I could live without you." I had usually just quipped, "Okay, dear, after you."

I didn't know how to get past the jokes and into the depths. Death talk had always been off limits in my growing up. That became especially clear one chilly evening when I was ten. My father drove the family to New York for dinner in a fancy restaurant followed by a Broadway musical. On the Henry Hudson Parkway, we inched past a car that had crashed and left an elderly man lying motionless on the pavement, his blue suit jacket and gray overcoat wide open, blood smeared on his face and white shirt. A knot of men stood around him, one of whom picked up a crushed gray hat from the pavement but, not knowing what to do with it, put it back down next to the man.

We all remained silent and still as my father jockeyed his way into the only lane with moving traffic, crept forward, and once past the accident, sped up fast enough to pin me against the back of my seat.

My mother, sitting tall and looking straight ahead, announced, "I'm sure he'll be fine."

Everything was fine. Death only happened someplace else.

* * *

By the time the issue arose of possibly talking with Jane about death, I'd already had four potential learning opportunities: my mom had died first—she was only forty-eight—then her mother, Gram, followed by my brother Al—he was fifty-four—and lastly my father. Strangely, though, my involvement in their deaths, subdued from the start, became even more so from one to the next.

I was twelve when my mom stopped Al and

me on our way out the front door. We were each wearing a New York Yankees cap and a baseball glove, mine filled with a hardball, Al toting a bat.

"I went to the doctor yesterday, and he found a little lump here," my mom said, pointing to her breast. I blanched. I had never before seen her point to her breast. "He's going to scoop it out, and I should be fine."

I didn't understand why she had a lump, how the doctor found it, or how he would remove it. But I didn't ask. I envisioned a melon ball scooper, a Band-Aid, and home for lunch. But it was many days and nights before she was home again.

Apparently scooping didn't provide a total cure. My parents took to calling her ailment arthritis, so for me that's what it was. It didn't occur to me to ask what arthritis had to do with her lump, her fatigue, or her radiation treatments. Eventually, though, she recovered her strength and remained healthy for several years. Arthritis cured, I assumed.

Once cured, she would sometimes spend whole days on her arts and crafts—not only printed art like wood cuts but also crafting fine wood furniture for our home. She also voluntarily presented a yearlong arts and crafts program at a hospital for physically disabled children. She never talked about those children, though, nor did she invite me to come to one of her craft lessons and meet them.

At about the time I went off to college, my mother's "arthritis" returned. During the summer following my junior year in college, I lived at home and had a summer laboratory job at the Albert Einstein College of Medicine in the Bronx. I became friends with two of the young doctors. I mentioned to them my mother's arthritis and asked a few questions regarding her treatment. They seemed reluctant to answer me.

One evening toward the end of the summer, I came home early and drove down the hill to the Hastings train station to pick up my father from his commute. Standing beside the car, I tried to pick him out from the long line of dark-suited men stepping from the platform up to street level. There he was in a dark blue suit, his tie loosened, the top button of his white shirt undone. He was holding the afternoon edition of the *New York Herald Tribune*, open to the stock page.

As I turned the ignition key, he pulled a crimson pack of Pall Malls from his shirt pocket and lit up, filling the car with smoke. I drove through town and turned up Edgars Lane, our hill, passing one lovely home after another. He started coughing, rolled down his window, and spat out a wad of phlegm. I pulled up to our long, steep stairway leading to our front door.

I turned off the engine, drew the key from the ignition, and reached for the door handle.

"Wait," my father blurted. "You know your mother is very ill."

"Yeah, arthritis. We've known that for years."

He shook his head. "It's cancer and she's dying."

With those five words—later, I fingered them out several times on my hand—he swung open his door, stepped out, threw his cigarette butt onto the sidewalk, snuffed it out with a swivel of his shoe, closed the car door, and tramped up the stairs to the house.

I knew he would go directly to the kitchen table for the dinner my mom was still able to prepare for us most nights. I was expected to be there too.

But I couldn't follow him.

I started pacing down Edgars Lane in the gathering darkness. The streetlights blinked on, blurring my teary vision.

How could I not have known? Me, a pre-med

major. Surrounded that summer by doctors I could have pressed for answers.

If I didn't show up for dinner, my mom would worry, so I soon turned around and trudged back up the hill.

In the kitchen, my parents had nearly finished their dinner. "So I told them," my father was saying, "I could get a full-color ad into half a million mailboxes within two weeks. And that really did it."

"Half a million! Can you really do that?"

"Of course I can, Bea—well, maybe three weeks—but the point is, that's when they signed."

"Good for you, Meyer."

Placing my dinner plate in front of me with her left hand, my mom leaned her right hand on my shoulder. I shrugged it off.

"What's the matter?" she asked.

"Nothing's the matter, right, Jeff?" my father broke in, glaring at me.

Nothing? Everything important was nothing. What I wanted was to lean on her; to depend on her, as I always had.

"Jeff, you'll do the dishes," my father declared, as he stood up and shuffled into the living room, then flipped on the TV news and lay down on the couch. My mom went upstairs to bed.

Over the sound of running water and clattering dishes, I heard from the broadcast something about space exploration. I turned the water down to a quiet drizzle. The familiar voice of Walter Cronkite was reminding viewers that fifteen months previously President Kennedy had declared that America would put a man on the moon by the end of the 1960s and that just six months ago John Glenn had become the first astronaut to orbit the earth. Now, on this day, the unmanned space probe Mariner 2 was setting off on its remarkable three-and-a-half-month journey to Venus. This was to be the first time a rocket would approach another planet, and it would transmit lots of information back to earth.

The thought of a rocket soaring out into the universe, freed from the pull of earth's gravity, then just flying effortlessly forward, gave my heart a thrill. Yet there, in my own small universe, as I sponged away the remains of our meatloaf, gravity weighed me down.

Cronkite concluded with his signature signoff, "And that's the way it is."

* * *

During my last year of college and first year of graduate school, I visited my parents in their apartment when I could. My sequential visits there felt like a series of snapshots of my mom's deterioration. Gladys, our once-a-week cleaner ever since I could remember, became my mom's daily caregiver.

On one of my visits, about two months after Jane's and my third wedding, my mom was sleeping soundly as I sat in the chair beside her bed. Her face was swollen from steroids, her graying hair disheveled, lipstick smudged in one corner of her mouth. Half completed *New York Times* crossword puzzles littered the bed.

She opened her eyes, smiled, reached out to clasp my hand, and murmured, "Jeff, I'm never going to get better."

She knew.

She wanted me to know.

She wanted me to know that she knew.

Exactly what she knew wasn't clear; but how could she not have known it was cancer? Sitting there with her, after years of silence, finally an opportunity to talk, listen, share—an opportunity, though, that threatened to take me to an unfamiliar, dark, and scary place.

I let go of her hand and replied flippantly: "Of course you're going to get better."

Those were the last words my mom and I ever spoke to each other about her illness. The word *death* was never mentioned.

The phone call arrived in Cambridge early one morning about a month later. My mother had died in the night. Jane and I drove down from Cambridge.

At the grave, we never saw the coffin, hidden under a bright green swath of Astroturf. The coffin descended electronically into the grave as if in a department store elevator.

Jane and I stayed behind after everyone had headed back to the parking lot.

I stood there for some time, immobile.

Then I began pacing, slowly, step by small step, full circle around my mom's grave.

One last embrace.

In silence.

* * *

A few years later, in Ithaca, I received a rare phone call from Al in his Connecticut home. "Is everything all right?" I asked. Yes, he assured me, and we chatted on about each other's work, our families, travel plans. Then he blurted out, "Oh, by the way, Gram died."

"What! When?" My maternal grandmother was old but had not been ill, as far as I knew.

"Oh, about two, no, maybe three weeks ago." He said it would have been hard for me to make it down for the funeral on Long Island, a full five-hours away by car. Al would later inform me, in similarly casual, after-the-fact calls, about the deaths of our maternal grandfather, two uncles, and two aunts. I came to accept, even appreciate, his tardiness. Not knowing when a relative was fatally ill meant no need to wonder what to say or to suffer the pain of a burial.

At some point, though, I was shocked at myself for accepting this pattern of death-hush. Had I insisted on being kept abreast of illnesses and deaths, this could have drawn me closer to the family and provided me with opportunities to mourn with them, to both feel and express compassion. Was I, the younger brother, considered too frail for all that? And if so, did repeated instances of such overprotection make me even more frail?

* * *

Years later, about a decade after our move to Jerusalem, I received a phone call from Al's son. We chatted idly until he said, "By the way, my dad's a bit sick, and we were wondering if you have any plans to visit sometime soon."

I was, in fact, due to give a lecture not far from their home, in less than a month.

"What's wrong with him?" I asked.

"Oh, it's a fever."

About an hour after that call, Jeremy rang me from Pennsylvania, where he was apprenticing in fine woodworking. Somehow, he knew about the phone call I'd just received.

"Dad, you'd better get over here right away." Al had been diagnosed half a year earlier with a fatal form of amyloidosis, a blood disease. "It's crazy," Jeremy said. "I've visited them three times in recent months and no one said a word until they phoned me just moments ago."

Al died the next day, ten minutes before I arrived. Later, in a moment of dark humor, I imagined that Al had arranged that timing so that he and I wouldn't have to talk about it.

Ellen and I hugged and cried as his shrouded body was carried down the stairs and out the door. Early images flipped through my mind: Al giving me batting practice, teaching me to ride a bicycle and later to drive a car, advising me about girls, about school, about college.

After the funeral, Ellen told me that Al felt he'd had a good life and was not troubled about its early termination. Not troubled—that was Al, all right. I half expected a phone call from his grave two or three weeks later to inform me, somewhere in a casual conversation, "By the way, I died."

* * *

Al's funeral was the last time I ever saw my father. He and I had been estranged for decades. Neither of us had explicitly declared the break; it just happened. For years there had been no visits, phone calls, or letters. Except one letter that I received rather early in our estrangement, when we were still living in Ithaca.

Back then, Saturday mornings were a key together time for Jane, seven-year-old Jeremy, and me, and we always gathered at the dining room table for a grander than usual breakfast. On this particular morning, I heard the mailman's footsteps on our front doorstep and a single thick envelope poked through the mail slot. The return address showed it to be from Meyer Camhi in Miami.

I tore it open and read its three pages.

Slowly.

Silently.

"What's the matter, Dad?" Jeremy asked.

I had assumed that my father's litany of anti-Jane accusations would fade with time, but there, on these pages, they had grown in number and fury. She was now "a witch who has turned you against the whole family. She's four years older than you and crafty—why can't you see that she finagled you into getting her pregnant?"

Jane and I tried later to laugh that one off.

"Finagling," we agreed, must be a lovemaking position we didn't know. Later, we would occasionally joke about it in bed: "I'm ready, dear, finagle me now," I would call out. But deep inside our laughs lay a core of pain. I buried his letter in my bedside drawer where it remained, forgotten, even after we, the bed, and the drawer moved from Ithaca to Jerusalem.

Over the years, I found myself trying to understand what had made my father the way he was. Although he had hardly shared any information with me about his early years, his brothers, Lou and Jack, had sometimes talked about their shared childhood. Their mother had died giving birth to Jack, the youngest, my father being the middle son. Their father, a low-grade worker in a traveling circus, couldn't—or wouldn't—raise his children and maintained no contact with them, so the three boys grew up together in an orphanage.

Lou and Jack both told me that when each of them had gotten married, my father had behaved despicably toward their brides. I also recalled that both before and for more than a year after Al and Ellen's wedding, my father had held Ellen in deep contempt and imposed the same silent treatment upon her that he later inflicted on Jane.

I came to believe that, having been "abandoned" by both his mother and father, he experienced the marriage of his brothers and, later, his sons as further abandonment, their brides stealing them from him. Not only was I the last to marry, but I also did so just as he was losing his wife.

One day, as I was mulling over what I knew about my father's early life, I wondered how he would have turned out if, as a little boy, someone like Jane had found him in the orphanage and adopted him—as she had found and we had adopted Alon. Not only how would he have turned out, but how would I?

In 2006, on my sixty-fifth birthday—three years before my retirement from the Hebrew University and our trip to Kyoto—Jane asked me, "Don't you want to know if your father is alive or dead? In good or bad health? Maybe even go see him?" She had asked a few times before, and my answer had always been no. But on this occasion, perhaps influenced by my own sense of aging, I decided it was time.

She suggested I do an online search for him. Not expecting much, I typed in his name followed by "Death Records, Florida," and almost instantly, his data popped up, including his accurate date of birth. He had died in 2005, aged ninety-two.

An unfamiliar numbness washed over me. Neither sadness nor disappointment at having missed him by just one year. Although his death brought to a close the many years of estrangement, it did not feel to me like closure.

The next day, I excavated his letter from my bedside drawer, recalling that for years I had been sleeping in between Jane and my father's letter vilifying her. I thought about Alon, Jeremy, Ariela, and my three grandchildren. What a loss my father had brought upon himself! He knew nothing of their lives or mine. Having grown up an orphan, he had then reorphaned himself.

Strangely, though, I felt as though his absence all those years had been a kind of gift. It had freed me from having to deal with his distressful loathing of Jane, with his old age and any accompanying illness or dementia, and finally, of course, with his death.

Jane entered the bedroom and I waved the three-page letter at her. "Remember this?"

She shook her head.

"It's the infamous finagle letter."

I expected a laugh or at least a smile. But she surprised me; "Jeff, we were at your mother's burial decades ago. Maybe now you can finally bury your father."

I took a deep breath.

Jane sat down beside me, her arms around my waist.

I held the three pages together between my thumbs and forefingers and slowly ripped the pages in half, then into quarters, then into many tiny pieces.

Jane squeezed my waist as I stared at the scraps of his life in my cupped hands.

I walked over to the empty, black wastebasket in the corner of the room and as I uncupped my hands, the scraps floated into the dark.

| 11 |

The Cure

About one and a half years had passed since Kyoto, and in the intervening months, Jane's sentences had become shorter, were occasionally incomplete, and often lacked any clear meaning. But one morning after finishing our oatmeal, as I carried in our coffee cups from the kitchen, she whispered, "Is there a cure for this?"

I plonked the cups on the table, splashing coffee right near her trembling hands. I edged my chair closer to hers and peered at her quivering lips.

"Is there a cure?" she repeated.

This simple sentence had several possible meanings:

"Jeff, I'm slipping; hold me."

"Jeff, I'm sinking; save me."

"Jeff, I'm scared; protect me."

I wanted to hug her or even to pick her up and rock her in my arms, as I had with Jeremy and with Alon as babies; to tell her, "I'm here with you always;" to admit, "I'm scared too." Determined to adhere to Dr. Ban's urging not to utter the word Alzheimer's for fear of plunging her into depression, I now considered lying in order to comfort her with the false hope of a cure.

What passed my lips, though, was something different. "A cure for what, Jane?"

How would she name it now? Always clever with words, she had first labeled it a natural condition, namely, her "aging brain," later shifting to a possibly curable ailment, her "brain disorder."

"A cure for what?" I asked again.

"My brain disintegration." Her voice crackled.

Those three words hit me like a sharp blow. Disintegration means crumbling. You don't get over crumbling. From crumbling you die. Did she know that?

"Would you like to talk about it?" I asked.

Would she?

Could I?

After some thought, she answered, "Not now."

Not ever, it turned out.

* * *

I was to replay that scene many times in my mind, wishing it had transpired like this:

"Is there a cure for this?" she asks.

I place a hand on her shoulder. "Well, let's talk about that, dear."

We look into each other's eyes. I lean in close and feel her warm breath washing over me.

"I'm part of your cure, you know."

She smiles, reaches for my free hand, and squeezes.

"For instance," I continue, "I know every inch of your back and which inches you most like me to scratch."

She squeezes tighter.

"And I know just how you like your oatmeal—banana slices, honey, and whole milk, not that feeble low-fat stuff that I drink."

She peeks into her bowl.

"And I know just how you like me to brush your hair."

She runs her fingers through her white curls, and her smile broadens.

"And when you smile as you're smiling now," I say, stroking her cheek, "I can feel your cure happening. So I guess I can say yes, there's a cure, and that cure is you and me."

"I love you, Jeff."

"And I love you too," I reply.

If only that scene had really happened.

PART III

ASCENT

| 12 |

Doors

It seemed almost predesigned that my very first hint of Jane's confusion, at the Kyoto T-junction, had occurred while we were celebrating my retirement—the closing of doors to my teaching and research. What higher force might have choreographed that just when Jane might start needing more of me, I would be more available, not running off to work early each morning and remaining there until early evening?

But Jane's need for more of my time didn't begin right at that T-junction moment; rather it developed gradually thereafter, a factor also seemingly predesigned to allow new doors to open for my postretirement era.

* * *

My first new activity was creating a new museum at the Hebrew University. It would consist mostly of permanent outdoor exhibits on the university's beautiful science campus, and its subjects would be nature and science. Not requiring a building would radically decrease the cost of creating and operating the museum. I proposed this project to the university authorities, and they approved it.

There was just one small problem: I knew nothing about how to create or manage a museum, whether indoors or out. So I began educating myself by extensive reading, attending international museum conferences, and visiting some of the world's great natural history museums and interviewing, where possible, their directors and key staff members. I began raising funds, hired some experienced staff, and recruited the voluntary assistance of faculty colleagues whose expertise encompassed the subjects of the planned exhibits. In time, we produced permanent exhibits about the trees on campus from all around the world, the birds that reside on campus and others that drop by during their semi-annual migrations, plant evolution, forest ecology, wildflowers, and scientific research on the campus.

By the time Jane had greater need of me, the museum was well along in development, and I could direct its operation at odd hours, leaving me time at home with her each day.

* * *

My second new activity entailed writing. Throughout my academic career, most of my published works had been technical and academic in both purpose and style. However, I had recently published a different sort of book. *A Dam in the River* was not technical and was not intended specifically for an academic audience. It analyzed the extent to which universities and colleges share their knowledge with the general public—a subject intimately connected to my museum work.

I thoroughly enjoyed writing *Dam* and wanted to go further and learn a broader range of writing styles and skills. So, I took writing courses, participated in relevant workshops, and joined a writers' group. While at first I didn't know why I was doing all that, I ultimately discovered that I was beginning to write *Care for the Carer*. Unlike my museum work, which took me to the university campus, I was most comfortable writing at home and was thus available in case Jane needed me.

* * *

At first, I successfully managed to split my time three ways: administering the campus museum, writing at home, and being with Jane. Later, though, Jane began wanting more of me, and although I loved my time with her, being together for hours, merely for the purpose of being together, felt burdensome. I got edgy. Cranky. If I declined her invitation, she would grumble, "Why are you always disappearing from me?" Jane seemed to be nudging my two newly open doors at least partly shut.

Unclear how to proceed with this problem and where to turn for advice, I scheduled a consultation with Dr. Ban. He pulled out a calling card from his file: "Dr. Adina Maeir, Professor of Occupational Therapy."

"She's good," he said. "She can help you."

I phoned and arranged an appointment in her home.

* * *

Wearing a floral blouse, jeans, sneakers, and a welcoming smile, Adina, who looked to be in her early forties, greeted me at her front door. She led me to her cozy office, whose walls displayed not advanced degree certificates but family photos, and whose desk exhibited not stacks of books and journals but a vase of freshly cut garden flowers. We sat opposite one another. A tissue protruded from the Kleenex box on the low table between us.

I wondered what kind of advice an occupational therapist would have to offer me. Her main expertise, I understood, was helping injured or physically disabled patients with motor skills. She'd be more relevant to Alon, I imagined.

At her request, I outlined the story of Jane's and my life together, focusing mostly on the time since Kyoto. I went on and on and was surprised when, glimpsing at my watch, the hour had flown by. I just managed to squeeze in that I was beginning to feel slightly trapped at home.

"If you like, we can set up a series of meetings to explore how you can take good care of yourself," she suggested.

"You mean of Jane," I corrected.

"Jane too, of course."

| 13 |

Something Good

One evening after my first several meetings with Adina, Jane sat next to me on our living room couch and pulled a printed notice from her pocket: "Reminder—next Aging & Saging meeting at my house Wednesday, 7:30 PM. Sue." Jane peered at it, perhaps to fix the time and place in her memory. That wasn't necessary, though, as I was keeping track of her A&S meetings, driving her to them, and picking her up afterward. She slid the notice back into her pocket. Every one of Jane's A&S meetings renewed my pride in her; she was its wellspring. Now, several years after she'd founded the discussion group, its members still regarded her as its honorary leader, despite her struggle to follow and participate in the conversation.

I switched on the TV to catch the evening

news. I might have searched for a good movie, but Jane was no longer able to follow the plot. She couldn't follow the newscast either, but she enjoyed watching the attractive broadcasters and their brief video clips.

When the news ended, Jane announced, "I have news."

Was she imitating the TV? Or did she really have something to say?

"No aging."

She pulled the notice back out of her pocket and placed it on my lap.

"They look at me … I can't." She began to cry.

I wrapped my hands around hers. Her hands that had typed that first memorable invitation five years earlier, initiating A&S and suggesting such discussion topics as "issues of life and death, significant turning points, definitive moments, our sense of self …"

Words that so epitomized Jane.

Words that she now could barely understand.

I lifted her hands to my lips and held them there for a long while, trying to ease her distress. And mine.

With the ending of something so fundamentally Jane as her role in A&S—something

so much a part of who she had been and what she had thought and cared about—I sensed her plummeting. And me with her.

* * *

When I arrived at Adina's for my next session, I must have looked dreadful. I explained Jane's decision about A&S and how deeply it pained me.

"I certainly can see your pain," she said, "but ..."

Why a "but?" I puzzled.

"But I'm thinking some good may come of this," she continued.

She mentioned that Jane had good, solid friends who cared about her, and surely her absence from A&S would be a great loss to them. Now maybe they could modify their way of being with her—caring not just about her, but for her. She suggested that I invite some of them over to visit Jane on a regular basis to help out.

Help out with what? I wondered. I had the shopping, cooking, cleaning, laundry, and errands all pretty much covered.

"They could just be with Jane. Read to her,

play a game with her, take her for a walk. Or a drive."

"Just a minute." I held up my hands as if to fend off her words. Take Jane for a drive? Kerouac Jane? Bad enough that she had given up her car keys and now A&S, but to be driven around like some decrepit old woman? I couldn't bear it; didn't even want to hear about it. Besides, I couldn't expect her friends, who were busy with their families and their jobs, to make regular visits.

"So you think Jane's best friends don't care about her?"

No answer.

She handed me a pad and a pen and asked me to list Jane's closest friends. Hesitantly, I dashed off three names—Naomi, Sue, and Rachel, all participants in A&S. I left off a few others, whose work or family obligations I knew to be especially heavy.

Then she asked about family. For instance, how often did Jeremy visit Jane?

I mentioned his Friday lunch visits.

"And what does he do when he comes for lunch?"

"He eats."

Adina said nothing.

I added Jeremy to the list.

"And Alon?" she asked.

She knew about Alon's disability, of course, and that he was cared for by Priyantha. How could Alon help Jane?

"Jane's disabled, too," Adina pointed out. "Alon might have a special sense of what that's like for her."

I gulped. She really got it about Alon. His name went straight onto the list.

"Who else?" Adina asked.

Ariela, Jeremy's wife. While Jeremy was always busy working, Ariela was free most days, and Jane loved her visits.

Adina didn't have to mention the grandchildren; I was already writing them down. Carmiel at age twenty-one was a soldier, Ortal, a high school senior, and Ishai, a tenth grader. Busy youngsters all, I didn't know how often they'd be free to visit.

Suddenly my cell phone rang. I looked at the screen.

"Jane again, third time this morning," I whispered to Adina.

"Hi, dear ... Glasses? Are they hanging around your neck?"

"Yes? Good."

"No, sorry, I can't come now. I have lots of work at the university today. I left you a nice lunch in the fridge."

"Yes, it's cold, but tonight I'll make us a nice hot dinner." Given the danger of Jane starting a fire or leaving the gas on, I turned off the stove's hidden gas valve whenever I finished cooking.

"See you later, dear. Goodbye."

Adina suggested I invite the people on my list to a meeting to discuss how they might contribute some time to care for Jane. Alon agreed to host the meeting, and I emailed invitations to eight people.

* * *

To my surprise, all eight showed up. Alon and Priyantha had set out some simple refreshments and arranged a circle of chairs with a space for Alon's wheelchair. I sat down next to him and thanked everyone for coming. Then I mentioned that perhaps they weren't all aware of how much Jane's condition had worsened.

I explained about the number of times a day she lost her glasses. About her inability to complete a simple sentence or to use the TV remote or even the toaster. I talked about the insects. Jane saw hundreds of them, thousands even, running around on the living room walls. To her, they were real, and she yelled at me for "pretending" I didn't see them—and me a biologist. She said that was really "pissy" of me.

My agitation must have shown, as Alon reached for my hand. "You know she doesn't mean it, Dad. Like you explained to me, it's her Alzheimer's talking, not her."

That calmed me down a bit.

The good news, I assured them, was that Jane still had her lovely smile and her hysterical laugh. Like when she would say something nonsensical and knew it and would then belt out a guffaw that would draw me in and we would sit there belly laughing together.

"I know you all love Jane's smiles and laughs, and that's why I thought maybe it's not too unfair of me to ask if you could visit her every now and again."

"You've got it all wrong, Jeff, " Naomi interrupted. "Unfair? It would be unfair of you not to ask for help." She added that Jane had always advised and comforted her, and she had long wanted to do something in return but hadn't wanted to intrude.

Several heads were nodding.

"And besides," Sue added, "with Aging and Saging probably disbanding—"

"What?" I retorted.

"Yes, didn't you know? Without Jane, it's just not the same. It looks like it's over."

I had hoped that A&S would continue and would be seen, to some extent, as Jane's legacy. But just ending like that, I was shocked. Five years of deep discussions turned to silence, just as Jane herself was becoming silent.

Those sitting with me in the circle must have sensed my dismay, as they stopped talking for a few moments to let me recover.

* * *

The first to resume talking was Sue, who offered to visit Jane once each week for a few hours. She said that during her visits, I should go and do whatever I wanted. "Jane will be covered, and you'll be free," she proclaimed.

Free? I sat there silently enjoying the sound of that word.

Rachel suggested that we make a schedule. She wrote down a day and time she would visit Jane each week, and everyone else followed suit, though our three grandchildren couldn't commit to specific days and times. And indeed, from then on, one or two friends or relatives visited Jane every weekday, each for a few hours.

Soon, a few more of Jane's friends signed on. One was Dianne, a music therapist. I was amazed how she drew Jane out, playing a song on her smartphone, giving Jane a tambourine or a xylophone or maracas and getting her to play and sing a few words.

And me? During those hours, I could write upstairs or drive to the university and work on some museum matter. I was gradually beginning to feel a little of what Sue must have meant by, "You'll be free."

* * *

On one occasion I headed upstairs to do some writing when Laura came over to read to Jane. Overworked as a professional tour guide, struggling to care for her six kids, and harried by divorce proceedings, she was unable to visit Jane regularly. I was amused that she had arrived carrying the Dr. Seuss book *Yertle the Turtle*, so I paused on the upstairs landing as she and Jane settled onto the living room couch. Laura's voice boomed out the story.

Jane made up a new name, "Turtle the Yertle," and Laura asked, "Do you think Yertle loves Myrtle?" Their laughter pealed right up the stairs to me.

When they'd finished the book, I went into the bedroom to work on my computer.

Yertle the Turtle made me smile.

"Turtle the Yertle" made me giggle.

"Does Myrtle love Yertle?" made me chuckle.

And then all these three made me cry.

Getaway

I had always loved going to concerts. So had Jane, and we had usually gone together. For several years, we had regularly attended a baroque ensemble, various jazz performances, and occasional concerts of the Israel Philharmonic. But this had ceased, as Jane could no longer sit still for more than a few minutes. Our musical experiences were reduced to my playing the piano for her, listening to a music station on the radio, or catching a performance on TV.

One evening after dinner, as we sat in the living room, I switched on the TV and found a lovely young pianist named Yuja Wang playing Chopin. I'd never heard of her. Her fingers flitted across the keyboard with such grace, her pianissimos so faint, fortissimos so bold. Her heart moved her hands, and her hands moved my heart. I drifted into a brief fantasy of sitting at a Yuja Wang concert, somewhere in the world—something that I knew, of course, wasn't going to happen.

But just a few days later, I opened the *Jerusalem Post* and wham, a full-page photo of Yuja Wang stared at me, advertising her forthcoming concert!

At the Jerusalem Convention Center!

Just a ten-minute walk from my house!

Jeremy agreed he would sit with Jane that evening.

I rushed to the ticket office.

"How many, sir?"

My voice cracked: "Just one."

* * *

Having found my seat in the concert hall, I glanced at the program. She was to begin with the Chopin Nocturne in E Flat Major. I had played that piece at a music competition when I was fifteen—of course nothing like the way she would play it. Sitting there, waiting for her to walk on stage, I fingered the nocturne's first few lines on my knees.

Yuja wafted onto the stage wearing a midnight-blue gown and looking even more lovely than she had on TV. She bowed deeply. Sitting at the keyboard, she leaned in gently as if caressing the piano, even as its curves caressed her. Her playing carried me away.

When I returned home, Jane was asleep on the couch, and Jeremy was sipping a beer in a nearby chair. When I asked how she had been, he replied okay, but she had asked where I was, and kept on asking, ultimately getting angry that I wasn't there with her.

Oh my! Maybe my going out had been a mistake. Maybe concerts or evening outings in general needed to be shelved. The next morning, though still humming Chopin, I had more or less concluded that, for Jane's sake, I should say no to outings intended for just my own pleasure.

* * *

In my next session with Adina, when I explained about Jane's reaction to my being out for a few evening hours, she surprised me by asking, "When did you last get away, not for a few hours, but for, say, a two- or three-day vacation?"

What a strange question. Didn't she understand how uncomfortable Jane would be traveling, staying in a hotel, and eating in restaurants?

"No, not you and Jane. Just you," she corrected.

What? Given Jane's response to my being at a concert for two hours, how could I possibly go away for two or three days? Who would keep her company, make her meals, put her to bed at night, be with her when she wakes in the morning and then all day long? She would be furious, and rightly so. Out of the question.

Adina didn't pursue the matter further during that meeting, but in our next session, she brought it up again. "What if you were to take yourself to a hotel in Tel Aviv for a few days?" She asked if I would enjoy the sea, a sauna, a stroll along the boardwalk, a massage.

I replied that I couldn't enjoy any of that while Jane sat alone at home.

She persisted, pointing out that I could arrange for all the people who visit Jane during the week to concentrate their visits on the days I'd be away and that Jeremy and Ariela could stay overnight with her.

I hadn't thought of that option.

But still, what if Jane got angry—furious

even—at my absence? That evening, though, I thought about the beach.

The sound of waves.

The mist in my face.

The freedom to do what I want, when I want, not for two hours, but for, say, two full days.

Maybe Jane would be happy to have all those people visiting.

A few days later, I picked up the phone and booked a room for one night in a five-star beach-front hotel in Tel Aviv.

* * *

I paused during a stroll in the early after-noon along the seaside boardwalk. Placing my elbows on the railing, I watched the waves blown in by the stiff breeze. Each wave exploded into a whitecap and its foam cooled my face. Just then, my cell phone rang.

"Where are you?"

"In Tel Aviv. Are you enjoying your visitors?"

"Tel Aviv, what the hell?"

"I told you I have a conference here." (A necessary fib, I told myself.)

"You have what?"

"A conference. Have Naomi and Sue gone

home yet? Did you enjoy your lunch? There's dinner in the fridge for you, Jeremy, and Ariela. They'll be there soon, and they'll warm it up and share it with you. And they are sleeping over tonight. Tomorrow the grandkids are coming to see you. I think you'll have a good time."

"Come home now."

But I said that I couldn't, that she would enjoy all her visitors, and that I missed her and I'd be back with her late tomorrow. I blew her a kiss and hung up.

I continued my walk along the boardwalk and into the park. Later, a delicious dinner with a fine wine, a peaceful night's sleep, a morning massage, and an early afternoon return home.

At my next meeting with Adina, I thanked her for the hotel idea and admitted how relaxing it had been. What's more, based on reports from Jane's visitors, except for her angry phone call to me, she seemed to have enjoyed the two days.

I nonetheless asked myself, was it really okay for me to have gone away just for my own pleasure?

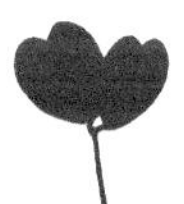

| 15 |

Lists

Late one afternoon, I headed out to the supermarket and bought several bottles of the pureed baby food that Jane was still able to eat without choking. Then to the pharmacy to refill her prescriptions—statins and thyroxin—and a department store to buy her two extra pairs of pajamas.

As I completed each purchase, I crossed it off my list on the little yellow pad that guided me through each day—my secret little guardian against chaos. In the two and a quarter years since Kyoto, I'd already used up several yellow pads.

The next morning, as I stirred our oatmeal on the stove, Jane sat at the breakfast table with a pen and a little yellow pad of her own. She appeared to jot down a few words and then covered them with her hand as she turned to look at me.

"What's that you're doing, dear?" I asked.

"My day. Writing," she said.

"Yes? What's up today?"

"Some stuff."

"What kind of stuff?"

No answer.

"So can I help?"

"No. Stuff."

"But—"

"Stop it!" she hollered, banging her fist several times hard on the table.

I had to hold myself back from hollering back. From banging my own fist. From saying things I knew I'd regret.

We ate our oatmeal in silence.

* * *

In my next session with Adina, I recounted how I'd been trying to help Jane, how she'd responded, and how that made me really angry.

Adina said nothing at first. Then, quietly, "Maybe Jane didn't need the kind of help that you were offering her."

"But she was floundering. She couldn't do it." Jane was stuck, and I was just trying to unstick her. Couldn't Adina see that?

"Yes," she replied, "but maybe Jane needed something else from you at that moment."

"What, I should have written down her day? That would have really ticked her off."

"Maybe at that moment, Jane just needed a hug."

I slumped against the back of the chair, a hand over my eyes. How blind I'd been.

Clearly, Jane had been imitating me, simply trying to write a few words.

Words, which had always been her forte.

She was trying to make the smallest of decisions about just one thing she might do that day.

For half a century, Jane's big decisions had given structure to our family life.

* * *

The next time Jane sat at the table trying to write on her yellow pad, I was washing the dishes.

She caught me looking at her over my shoulder.

Again she banged the table.

I turned off the tap, dried my hands, and walked over to her.

"Jane, will you please stand up for a moment?"

With a suspicious tilt of her head, she pressed her palms firmly on the table, slowly lifting herself up. I stepped closer and wrapped my arms around her waist. Hesitantly, she placed her arms around my neck. I pulled her in close. We held each other tight, in silence, for a very long time, cheek against warm cheek, inhaling each other's scent.

I wanted to keep her from slipping out of my life.

I wanted to squeeze the Alzheimer's right out of her.

I wanted us to be who we once were.

None of that could happen.

But at least, from that day on, when words alluded Jane, hugs took their place.

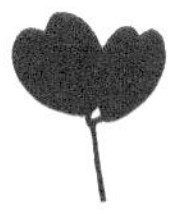

| 16 |

A Little Dance

I had already prepared a tofu salad for Jeremy and me, soft boiled eggs for Jane, and a carrot soup for all three of us. It was Friday, and lunchtime was approaching.

My cell phone rang. "Hi, Dad, I'm on my way … but I might not be such great company today."

A twinge shot down my neck. "Not such great company" could mean only one thing—money. Having trained as a fine woodworker in the States, he had become outstanding in the field. But he hadn't yet become outstanding in marketing his lovely works.

"We'll talk about it when you get here."

Damn, why did I say that? Jeremy was supposed to be coming to spend time with Jane.

When he arrived, we sat down for lunch, and I passed around the soup bowls. Jeremy leaned way back in his chair, stretched his arms forward, and fingered the edge of his bowl. He took a deep breath and exhaled with a mournful whisper, "I'm eighty-five thousand shekels in debt."

"Let's see," I mumbled, "that's about—"

"It's twen-ty-three-thou-sand-dol-lars, Dad!" he wailed, the palms of both his hands thumping the table.

I glanced at Jane, worried he might have startled her. But she was focused on directing a soup spoon to her mouth.

Jeremy started detailing his cash inflow and outflow. But very soon I tuned out, my thoughts wandering in a different direction. I realized that with Ariela being markedly deaf and not working, and Jane retreating more and more into her own world, I might be Jeremy's main— perhaps his only—address for his periodic panics about money.

Jane stood up, took a few steps toward her room, and stopped. She raised a hand to her forehead, seeming unsure where she was going, turned back to her chair, and pushed it in to the table, then turned toward the bathroom, entered, and closed the door behind her.

Jeremy shoved his chair back, shot up, and stomped into the living room, slamming his fists against his thighs.

What was going on? Was he just at that moment grasping what we were dealing with? What I was dealing with? What had he thought all those other Fridays when he came to visit? Maybe it was my fault—I'd never sat him down and detailed what life had become for Jane and me. But couldn't he see it? Or at least imagine it?

Having finished lunch, I surprised both Jeremy and myself by announcing that the two of us were going for a walk. I kissed Jane's forehead and told her we'd be back in soon. I knew I needed to speak with Jeremy, though I had no idea what to say or how to say it.

* * *

We walked in silence up a steep hill toward a small, empty park and sat on a bench shaded by an olive tree. Ill-formed thoughts jostled through my mind.

"I know it's a hard time for you now, Jeremy, with your overdraft. And I guess you're also starting to see just how disabled Mom is becoming."

He turned a blank expression toward me.

I reached over and held his arm.

I repeated something I'd said before, that if

he wanted some money he should just ask, and if I could help I would. But he shook his head, explaining, as he always had, that he didn't want my money.

"Well, in that case," I continued, "I can't help you. I really can't, Jeremy."

I suggested that he rely more on Ariela for sharing his money troubles. Maybe he should get a financial advisor, sell his house and move into an apartment, or do whatever people do when they're financially stressed.

"But as I'm sure you can see, my hands are full with your mom, and they're getting fuller by the day. It's all that I can handle, and I simply can't help you."

Never before had I told him anything like "I can't help you." Never before had I abrogated what I had always regarded as my parental responsibility. And now, as those words left my lips, I expected to feel distraught of saying them—ashamed at myself. But I was astonished to feel very different—relieved and even a bit lighthearted.

But there was more I needed to say.

"I'm just now figuring out why I can't help you. I think it's because I'm the one who needs help!" I paused to take in what I had just said. "Yeah, me, your dad. I need help."

With that, I stood up and, of all things, started singing, "I need help, I need help, I need help, help, help," softly at first then louder, and I started dancing to my tune, on and on.

Jeremy stood up and grabbed my arm, his wide-open eyes reflecting fear. "Dad, are you okay?"

"Yes. No. Okay? Jeremy, it's not just your mom who needs help." I went on with my little dance.

"Dad, what's the matter with you?"

"The matter? Nothing. And yet everything. I'm so happy. I'm so sad. Dancing, that's what I need," and I recalled dancing with Jane on that night way back when we had just moved into our newly purchased Ithaca home. Then I was celebrating our new home; now, a new realization.

He tried to laugh and even dance along with me, and there we were for that moment, father and son, prancing around together in the park.

My cell phone cut us short.

"It's your mom calling," I whispered, surprised; she usually couldn't remember how to use her cell phone.

"Okay, I will," I told her and hung up. "She wants me to get home now."

"Why?"

"She said, 'Where the hell is my book?'"

"But, Dad, she can't read anymore."

"I know. But she likes to think she can."

Jeremy stopped moving altogether. He looked straight at me and said, "Dad, I always thought you could do everything. I've never understood how, just that you could."

"But I can't, and if any more weight falls on my shoulders, I'll collapse. So you'll have to handle your work problems without me. From now on, I'm a dancer."

"I love that you dance, Dad."

"Good. I'm going to stay here for a few more minutes and remember how I used to feel when I danced. You go home and look for Mom's book. Okay?"

He did.

* * *

Later that day, I drove over to see Alon, part of my regular Friday routine. On the way, my cell phone rang, and I pulled over to answer.

"When are you coming?" There was urgency in Alon's voice. And the sound of a stuffed nose.

"I'm driving now. Can't talk. See you in five."

Can't talk? Didn't want to talk was more

like it. It was something about the sound of his stuffed nose.

I flashed way back to an incident when he was just two years old and clogged up. But then it wasn't mucus in his nostrils, rather, a blockage of the millimeters-narrow shunt tube implanted in his fluid-filled brain cavities. With the tube blocked, his cavities had been expanding with accumulating fluid and that was putting pressure on his brain. It called for emergency surgery to either flush out the tube or replace it.

I'd had a severe tension headache when that happened, and now, just thinking about it, my head ached again as I knocked on his door. Seated in his wheelchair, he opened the door, as it was Priyantha's day off. I sank into his couch, hoping that resting would relieve my pain.

Alon's face was red and sweaty. Crumpled tissues littered his lap.

"Got a cold," he said, "kind of bad."

He had tried to reach Dr. Ban, but he had already gone home.

"What should we do, Dad?"

I thought through our options. I could drive him to the twenty-four-hour emergency clinic. No need to phone Priyantha; I could lift Alon into the car and his wheelchair into the trunk. If things got really bad, there was the emergency room at Hadassah Hospital.

I asked if he had a fever.

No.

Sore throat?

A bit.

Coughing?

He nodded.

I tried massaging my neck and forehead. My mind drifted back to the first of Alon's various blocked shunt incidents that had required surgery. As we waited for an operating room to free up, the only thing that would relieve the pain in Alon's head, at least partially, was my carrying him back and forth along the hospital corridor, his forehead leaning on my shoulder. But on that day, a multicar collision had filled the operating rooms. So I walked on and on, hour after hour, his arm wrapped around my neck, his aching head on my shoulder, my head absorbing some of his pain.

But now I caught hold of myself. This current ailment is just a stuffed nose, for God's sake. Just a simple cold. I was shocked by my overreaction.

"Listen, Alon, I need to explain something that just happened to me."

"When?"

"Just now. In my head. I just figured out something about your very first shunt surgery."

"Dad, that was over twenty-five years ago."

I explained that, nevertheless, ever since that first of his medical emergencies, whenever he got sick, I would slip into worry mode and immediately start planning our best move. But now I'd suddenly realized the difference. "A blocked shunt sends us straight to the hospital. A crumpled Kleenex doesn't."

"Obviously, Dad."

I explained that it wasn't always so obvious to me, especially now that his mother was unable to help calm me down.

"Yeah, okay, but what are we going to do about my cold?"

I took a deep breath. I reminded him that whenever he had a real emergency, I was there with him, 100 percent, and always would be.

"Sure, Dad."

"But when you have a minor problem—and this cold of yours is a minor problem, as I'm sure you know—you don't need me."

I took another deep breath.

"And I have just started to realize that, given what's going on with your mom, I need you to keep me out of your minor problems so they don't weigh me down."

We both went silent for some time.

Then I added, "So from now on, when you have a simple cold or flu, Alon, it's *your* cold or flu and not ours."

I reminded him that he knew his medical options better than I did. He had taken a first-aid and CPR course, and he was very well acquainted with the layout of Jerusalem's medical system. He had volunteered for ten years at a medical assistance organization with numerous experts of all kinds. He had many friends working at Hadassah Hospital, and, of course, he had Dr. Ban. And Priyantha—even on his day off, a phone call would bring him right back.

Alon sat deep in thought. "So you don't want me to tell you when I have a cold?"

"Well, let's see. If you ask me on the phone how I am and I have a cold, I might say, 'Fine, except for this darned cold,' and you might say, 'Hope you get over it soon.' That's how we both should be about our colds and other cold-like stuff."

Alon was silent again. Then, "I'm sorry, Dad.

I guess I hadn't realized how hard this is for you, with Mom and all. This will take me some time to get used to. But I can do it." He looked up at me. "And I will."

When it came time for me to leave, my headache seemed to have almost disappeared. By the time I stepped outside his building, it was completely gone. I walked toward my car with a spring in my step. By the time I reached the car, that spring had almost transformed into a little dance.

Full House

"Jeff, I think it's great how you're managing," Adina announced at the start of a session.

This, I knew, was an opening line for presenting me with a new challenge. But as most of her challenges worked out well, I was listening.

"I'm thinking it may be time to add one more to those living in your house."

I shook my head. I'd heard this idea before from my men's group. They'd been urging me to hire a caregiving helper. I had sidestepped their suggestion, just as I did Adina's, replying, "Yes, I agree, it's time for us to get a dog."

I was only half joking. Jane had been pleading over and over for a dog. So far, I had objected—I didn't want dog-walking several times a day added to my list of chores.

I reminded Adina that I could handle the caregiving myself.

"So tell me, what can you handle?" she probed.

I reeled off my list: shopping, cooking, serving, dishwashing, running errands.

"Is that it?"

I added laundry and some house cleaning.

"That's great. But can you also handle showering Jane? Changing her diaper? Lifting her in and out of her wheelchair?"

What was she talking about? Jane took her own showers. She didn't wear diapers or use a wheelchair.

"Not yet."

That was right. Not yet. I suggested we delay this topic until it became relevant.

A long pause ensued.

Adina then asked me to describe a typical scene at our dinner table.

I took a deep breath. "We talk."

She asked what about.

Another deep breath. "About whether she wants some more cottage cheese."

Did we have insurance coverage for a live-in caregiver?

"Of course not."

She therefore suggested hiring someone for a few hours every day. That, combined with the ongoing daily visits from friends and family could relieve me, say, from after breakfast until midafternoon. During that time, I could go to the university and work on the museum or sit upstairs at my computer and write. Or just go for a walk, with or without friends. And then during my reduced time with Jane, I could be more fully with her.

Late that night, I recalled that, long ago, Jane had investigated a program for hiring a live-in foreign caregiver through Israel's National Insurance program. She had gotten really excited about the program and commented that one never knows what will be needed later on. We signed on then for coverage of one live-in caregiver.

But now, contemplating a foreigner living with us, I imagined someone with limited English. I'd have to constantly translate. Jane might find the language barrier problematic.

Of course, Jane herself now had only minimal English. But she and I had developed our own private language beyond words—the look in our eyes, the touch of our hands, our posture. And we had music—I played songs for

her on the piano, and sometimes she remembered a few of the words and sang them.

I put the caregiving issue on hold. For now,
caring for Jane was my job, along with the
much-appreciated help of friends and family.

* * *

Some days later, I made a simple dinner
for the two of us—soft boiled eggs with cottage
cheese, plus apple sauce for dessert. I mixed a
bit of cottage cheese into eggs for Jane, salted
lightly, half-filled a teaspoon, and handed it to
her. But she didn't take it. I placed the spoon in
her bowl, prepared my own egg and cheese, and
took a spoonful.

"Mmm, it's good. Try it," I urged.

She didn't.

I lifted her spoon toward her lips.

She scrutinized it.

I pressed it against her lower lip.

Her mouth remained stubbornly shut.

I pushed a little harder.

Why wouldn't she open?

Finally, her lips separated just enough for me
to angle the spoon upward, spilling its contents
onto her tongue.

"You can swallow now, Jane," I said, and she rolled her eyes as though I'd said something stupid.

"Go ahead and swallow," I repeated, beginning to feel edgy. It seemed like forever until she did. "Good, huh?" She nodded. Then another spoonful and another forever-pause until she opened.

The next morning, I contacted National Insurance, obtained an application for a foreign worker, and filled it out. It was three and a half years since Kyoto, and I needed help.

* * *

A few weeks later, a gray-haired, slightly plump doctor with a pleasant smile and a scruffy brown briefcase came to our house from National Insurance to "interview" Jane. Based on her level of disability, he would judge whether to approve our request for funding of a caregiver. He took a one-page form from his briefcase and began reading out a series of questions to me, recognizing that Jane was unable to answer. Less than halfway down the page, he looked my way: "No question about it, your request is approved."

In another few weeks, a document arrived in the mail. I was surprised to read, "Two live-in helpers approved."

That jogged my memory. When we'd purchased the insurance, there was an option for a second helper via the Hebrew University. Two helpers for Jane could work together, and the double insurance would cover nearly the full cost.

We'll start with just one, I told myself. I arranged for candidates to come to the house, one at a time, to interview for the position.

On the morning of the first interview, Jane waited on the living room couch, still in her pajamas but wearing a pretty silk scarf I hadn't seen in months, and lipstick, which I hadn't seen in years.

She arrived right on time, an attractive woman around thirty, short but sturdy and appearing confident but not overly so.

"Hello, I'm Armeda." She sat down next to Jane and reached for her frail, bony hand, its blue veins wrapped in tracing-paper skin. "You must be Jane. Nice to meet you."

Jane looked straight ahead. "Why are you here?"

"I thought maybe I be your friend. And maybe sometime I help you."

Jane straightened up and seemed to go rigid, looking slightly upward, her gaze fixed as if on some distant site. It was a look I knew well, from that Annapurna photograph on my piano.

"I don't need help," she replied.

Armeda pulled her cell phone from her pocket and asked Jane if she'd like to see a picture of her family—her husband and three kids.

Jane leaned toward the phone. "They're pretty. Who's this one?" she asked, pointing at the screen.

"Which one?"

Jane placed one hand under Armeda's, lifting the phone closer, and pointed again.

"Oh, that our dog." She laughed. "My husband's dog. He call dog Joe."

"Joe," Jane repeated, glancing over at me.

I asked where her family was.

"They back in Philippines," Armeda replied matter-of-factly.

"Joe. I like him," Jane said.

I suggested that Armeda tell us some of the ways she could help in the house.

Looking at Jane, she asked, "You like to eat? I can cook. I make nice soup. My main dishes okay but need more practice." She gave a little laugh, and Jane laughed with her.

"I think I like you, Jane," Armeda declared.

"I like you," Jane responded. "And Joe."

Impressed by the way Armeda made that connection, I imagined she must have had professional training, maybe as a nurse or a social worker. I asked her what her job was before she came to Israel.

"Fish," she replied.

"Fish?"

She explained that they lived near the sea. She would buy fish when the boats came in, pack them in ice, put them in her bicycle basket, and ride over the hill to an inland town. She would sell the fish there and then ride home.

I said that sounded like hard work.

She shrugged, "Not so bad. But money?" She wagged her head. That was why she'd come to Israel, she said, and why she sent the money earned back home. "I come for future of my children."

I leaned back and contemplated: would I have the strength to leave my family for several years, "for the sake of my children?"

She explained that she was looking for a new position because her previous employer, an elderly woman she'd worked with for years, had recently died.

She mentioned that she liked to go to church; it made her feel good. She would need time off for that. No problem, I assured her, and invited her to look around the house with me. I showed her the little guest suite that would be hers and sensed it was more than she had expected.

When we went back to Jane, she and Armeda held hands as I closed the deal.

She got up to go, saying she would come back tomorrow with her things. "Shalom, Jane," she said, and was gone.

The next evening, I discovered that Armeda could, in fact, cook a main course as delicious as her soups. She had made a separate main dish for Jane that was soft and smooth. Jane ate it with hardly any help from Armeda. Showing off, I suspected.

* * *

"Show me Joe," Jane pressed Armeda, several times a day. *Dog* had become one of

Jane's favorite words, as in, "We need a dog," or "Let's get a dog."

When Armeda agreed to be both a caregiver and dog walker, I drove with Jane to the SPCA.

I told the man in charge that we wanted a small, easygoing dog.

"And cute," Jane threw in.

He brought out a Pekingese.

Jane frowned. I guess she didn't think he was cute.

Next, he brought out a sweet, fairly small, floppy-eared mutt, probably part beagle, with short brown hair. It held its left rear leg in the air and walked on the other three.

"What's wrong?" Jane asked.

It was a broken leg, though not clear how it had happened; maybe hit by a car, he offered, adding that the previous owner just brought him and left without an explanation.

"Poor dog; cute dog," Jane said, bending down and scratching him behind his floppy ears. He turned his head and licked her hand.

"What's his name?" I asked.

"Golani."

"Golani." I laughed—like the Israeli Army's Golani brigade.

The man attached a leash to the dog's collar

and handed it to me, and we took him for a stroll around the grounds.

"I like him," Jane said.

"I think he likes you too," I told her. She flashed me a broad smile. That, for me, was the decisive moment.

We signed some papers, and the man carried a small, padded dog bed and bag of dog food to our car. Golani jumped in through the car's back door and onto the seat, all with just three legs. A brave soldier, I thought. Jane and I got into the front. As I started the engine with our new family member panting behind, Jane leaned over and, without any words, kissed my cheek. It was like her kiss, also in the car, also silent, when we first decided to adopt Alon.

* * *

"Ouch! Piss, piss!" Jane called out in the dark, waking me up.

"What's going on?" I reached over and felt her side of the bed. Empty. "Where are you?"

"My head. This door thing. Piss!"

"What are you doing over by the stairs?"

"Golani. Crying."

An electric charge shot through me. If she

tried walking downstairs in the dark, she could fall.

I encouraged Jane to come back to bed and I would run down and check out Golani who, anyway, was no longer crying. She agreed.

In the morning, I discussed with Armeda what had happened, and we decided that a new sleeping arrangement was called for immediately. Jane's study downstairs, just off the dining room, which had originally been Jeremy's bedroom and then Alon's, would now become Jane's bedroom. Armeda rearranged it for her that very day.

That evening, not knowing how Jane would take to the new arrangement, I put my arm around her shoulder. "You've got a whole new place to sleep tonight, dear. Look."

Armeda had made up the bed with brightly colored sheets. She had put a vase of freshly cut flowers on the desk and moved some of Jane's clothes onto the open shelves. "And Armeda will sleep here with you on the pullout bed."

Jane smiled, walked over, and puffed up her pillow.

"And maybe Golani come and visit us," Armeda added, which made Jane smile.

While Armeda got Jane ready for bed, I sat

in the living room, trying to read the day's *Jerusalem Post*.

All I could think of was Jane moving downstairs.

I knew it was the right thing to do.

But after nearly fifty years of sleeping together, Jane was leaving me.

My nights of holding her as we drifted off to sleep, of wrapping my arm around her waist, pressing my cheek against her warm shoulder, listening to her breathe in her sleep—all those were over.

When Armeda turned off the light in her room, I walked over to her bed. "Goodnight, dear," I said, kissed her forehead, and walked toward the door.

"Come, Golani," she called.

* * *

Armeda was working a twenty-four-hour shift, sleeping in Jane's room at night, waking whenever Jane did, and caring for her during the day. She rarely retreated to her own room or went out with friends, except to attend church. Though she never complained, it was clear I needed to find a second helper and provide Armeda with some relief.

I contacted the National Insurance again, and after a few interviews, Eunice, also from the Philippines, joined our household.

A few days later, when I heard a hubbub coming from the kitchen, I popped in to see what was happening. There was Armeda, chopping vegetables and chattering away in a mixture of Filipino and English, Eunice scrambling eggs while listening and giggling, Jane erratically spooning Ben and Jerry's vanilla ice cream to her lips and wearing a happy smile, Golani barking at Jane for a handout, and Celine Dion belting out from the radio, "My Heart Will Go On."

I took Jane's hand, placing her spoon on the counter, and invited her to stand up. I put my hand around her waist, and we began dancing around our kitchen with our helpers chopping, scrambling, and chatting, Golani chasing our feet, and roars of laughter intermingling with the music.

| 18 |

Lunch

"Have you ever considered joining a writers' group or having a writing partner?" Adina asked me.

I explained that I had been a member of a writer's group for quite a while, but it had recently disbanded. Given how much I had enjoyed it, I answered that I would be interested in a new group, or perhaps a partner.

Later that day, I searched online for writers' groups in Jerusalem. There were poetry groups, women writers' groups, writers of religious works, and more, some in Hebrew, a few in English. I found one that seemed suitable, but the person I phoned said the group was full.

Then I recalled that our friend Laura wrote both poetry and a personal journal. I had never read her work, but she, Jane, and I had long shared several common interests, so I thought she might be suitable. But Laura had her hands full at work and at home and was unlikely to be looking for additional commitments. Nevertheless, I made a note on my calendar to call her the following week. Anyway, we hadn't spoken in months; it would be a chance to catch up.

Two days later, my phone rang. It was Laura.

"Wow, this is spooky," I exclaimed, mentioning how I'd planned to phone her.

After a bit of chatting, she commented on how hard it must be for me at home now. She added that she also was going through a hard time and suggested we get together and talk about it, that it might be helpful for both of us.

I agreed and threw in the idea of a writing partnership. She confirmed what I already knew: she was very busy. Nevertheless, she liked the idea in principle.

I suggested lunch.

*　*　*

I arrived first at the terrace restaurant in the Jerusalem Botanical Garden and soon spotted Laura on the path bordering the swan pond. Lanky and graceful as a swan herself, she'd woven her long brown hair in a braid and wore a flowery blouse, beige pants, and sandals. She settled into a chair and wiped her brow and neck with her napkin, explaining that she'd cycled there, a twenty-minute ride. A delicate gold necklace gleamed against her tanned skin, complimenting her modest gold earrings. Her lips wore a touch of rose red.

We began catching up, her kids and mine, her work and mine.

When our salads arrived, I turned the conversation around to writing: what time of day did we each like to write? How many hours a day? By hand or on the computer? We chatted easily about these matters, but when I tried to deepen the conversation, asking how her ongoing divorce might be affecting her poetry or journal writing, she was reticent. Strange, I thought, as she had suggested that talking about our hard times might be helpful. Nevertheless, as we got up to leave, I asked if she'd like to meet again, and she nodded.

A few weeks later, sitting across from each other at a narrow table in a university coffee shop, we struggled to hear one another over the recorded music and the buzz of surrounding conversations.

"You know," Laura began, "living alone again now after twenty-seven years ..."

I pulled in my chair to hear better.

Our knees touched.

"It's good to be free of constraints, at least partially," she continued. "There were some really difficult ones all through my marriage. But it's strange; even living on my own now, I still feel partly constrained. You don't just flip a switch and feel free," she clarified. "You have to learn freedom to earn freedom."

I liked the rhyme.

"And the learning is hard," she continued. "First, I have to unlearn old ways, which sometimes feels even harder than learning new ones."

"You seem to be telling *my* story," I responded, "about unlearning and learning." I reached out, and we touched hands momentarily.

"Are you writing about this?" she asked. "Maybe I could read something of yours?"

"Yes, and maybe you could show me some of your poems?"

She nodded.

* * *

That night, beneath my covers, I started imagining what it might be like, Laura and me.

Forget it, I told myself.

I'm married.

Well, married officially though not functionally. Jane and I still talked, though our sentences averaged about four words in length. We still touched, though it was mostly me doing the touching. I could hardly remember how it was to feel truly married: when our meandering conversations would sometimes go on and on, when touching was our language of love, when we were two functioning adults.

But Laura and me? That seemed unlikely, me a senior citizen and she sixteen years my junior.

Me overweight and out of shape and she a trim and keen cyclist.

Me swallowing seven pills a day and she occasionally sucking a mint.

And then there was sex; me partially incapacitated like roughly half the men my age and she, I imagined, fully functional.

My thoughts rambled on.

I rolled over and scolded myself.

Laura was not an option.

* * *

I drove over to Laura's place one morning after her kids were off to school. We sat in her garden and talked.

About a week later, on the couch in her sunlit living room, we touched.

Late-night phone calls.

A few weeks later, we drove to Tel Aviv, rented bicycles, cycled on the boardwalk, ordered martinis and dinner at a beachside restaurant, and then settled in for the night at a nearby hotel.

I woke up at five. Laura opened her eyes briefly, laid her head and arm on my bare chest, and went back to sleep. I stayed awake listening to her breath, feeling her warmth.

When we were both up and dressed for breakfast, I held her and said, "With you so close to me this morning, I felt …" but I faltered, unable to find just the right word. I found it later, though, over breakfast. "With you so close to me this morning, I felt *whole*." I hadn't fully realized until then that I'd been living only part of life. Like Jane, in a sense. As she had been losing parts of herself, so had I.

Laura reached out and touched my hand. It felt like a lifeline.

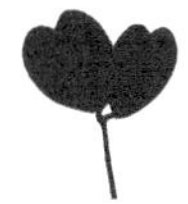

| 19 |

The Visit

"Jeff, I think dinner at your and Jane's place would be okay," Laura said.

She reminded me how she and Jane had been friends for thirty years and how she'd been to our home for Shabbat dinners so many times in the past. It was natural for that to continue, she suggested.

But I could see nothing natural about the idea of my sitting between Laura and Jane at our Shabbat table.

Laura understood but felt confident it would go smoothly. Jane might not even know who she was; that's how it had seemed during her most recent visit.

Four and a half years now since Kyoto, there was so little left of all that was once Jane. How would I feel now, how should I act, and how could I cope with sitting between the shadow of Jane and the fullness of Laura? I didn't know, but I put my trust in Laura's intuition.

* * *

Armeda and Eunice had set the traditional Shabbat table with places for the three of us and the two of them. They helped Jane light the Shabbat candles on the counter. Then, "Jane dear, you sit here," Armeda said, settling her into a chair. "And you're over there," she said, motioning to Laura.

I took my place between them at the head of the table.

Our silver kiddush cup was in front of me, ready for the traditional blessing over wine.

"Look, Jane," I said, lifting it toward her, "your grandfather's kiddush cup. See his engraved initials, CW?"

She didn't respond.

In the center of the table, two braided challah loaves beneath a beautifully woven cloth cover that Jane had bought years before at a workshop for the aged.

"Look, Jane, remember your challah cover?"

Again, silence.

The table was set with our good dinner

service: cream-colored stoneware that Jane and I had bought in Oxford during my first sabbatical leave from Cornell and the sterling silverware we had received as a wedding gift. The table reflected fifty years of Jane and me.

I filled the kiddush cup with wine, stood, recited the blessing, then sat down, pouring from this cup into four smaller silver ones and passing these around. My pinky brushed Laura's as I passed the little cup from my hand to hers.

Jane had always been the one to say the blessing over the challah. As she was no longer able, I invited Laura. After making the blessing, she cut several slices, sprinkled them with salt as is traditional, and passed them around.

"Jane, do you remember our long walks together," Laura asked, "when you were getting ready for Annapurna?"

Jane looked upward in silence.

"I miss those walks," Laura continued. "Maybe we could go for a short walk together sometime."

There seemed to be some kind of reaction on Jane's face, but I couldn't read it. Maybe she was trying to recall their walks? Or recall who Laura was and why she was sitting there?

Eunice served everyone soup and then pulled her chair close to Jane's to feed her.

As I tasted my soup, I started to feel an incipient pain right down my middle, as though Jane and Laura were two tectonic plates within me that were pulling apart and leaving behind a deep, aching chasm.

I looked over at Jane, who was sitting quietly, the trace of a smile on her face, and I realized that I was the one who'd been trying to reach out to her, pulling her in toward me with her grandfather's cup and her challah cover. I looked over at Laura, and it was the same: I had been reaching out to her, maneuvering my pinky to brush against hers, inviting her to say the blessing over the bread. I was, in fact, drawing the two women I loved toward me, into me, filling that chasm and, it seemed, creating within myself a state of wholeness.

* * *

After dinner, when Laura had left and Armeda had settled Jane into bed, I sat on the bed's edge.

"Did you enjoy the dinner with Laura?" I asked.

"Dinner."
"Did you enjoy it?"
"Yes."
She closed her eyes.
"With Laura?" I asked.
She opened her eyes, but for just a moment.
Soon she was asleep.

| 20 |

Going Public

Laura and I kept our relationship secret for a long while. But ultimately, we felt we ought to tell our kids. We decided we would each inform our own kids on the same day. That way, they'd all hear it directly from us and not from each other.

When I mentioned that I had some news to share, Jeremy and Ariela invited Alon and me to a family dinner at their house. Jane stayed home, of course, with Armeda and Eunice. I picked up Alon, and we drove there together. During the ride, he kept asking me about my news, so I had to keep changing the subject.

On arriving, I handed Jeremy a bottle of good red wine.

He thanked me and added, "Whatever your news is, I'm guessing this bottle will help us smooth out any rough edges." Interesting, I thought, that he predicted rough edges. I envisioned him sweating while sanding the edges of one of his wood creations.

In the kitchen, a delicious fragrance emanated from a large pot bubbling on the stove. I guessed spaghetti sauce. When the meal was ready, I made my way to the dining table, taking in the various items of beautiful wood furniture that Jeremy had made for their home—the freestanding shelf and cabinet unit, the armed lounge chair, and the dining table itself. Once we were all seated, my granddaughters, Carmiel and Ortal, served everyone spaghetti and meatballs and passed around a salad while their younger brother, Ishai, uncorked the wine. I sat beside Alon and opposite Jeremy.

"So are you giving us good news or bad?" Alon pressed, angling his wheelchair close to me.

"You'll decide," I said as I ran my arm across his shoulder and tugged him toward me.

"Something new about Mom's condition?"

"Not really."

Jeremy walked around the table, filling everyone's wine glass. Back in his chair, he called out, "L'chaim," and, as we all sipped, he turned to me. "Okay, Dad, you're on."

* * *

Slowly, and with a touch of the histrionic—permissible at my age, I told myself—I lifted my wine glass and took a long, slow sip.

"Umm, Dad, you're on," Jeremy repeated.

"Suppose you owned a big, beautiful wine goblet," I began, "far more ornate than the one in my hand."

"What? You don't like our IKEA glasses?" Ishai quipped.

I continued, describing a goblet of many colors and the highest quality crystal perched atop a long, thin stem.

"You're going all dramatic on us, Dad," Jeremy interrupted, "and you've hardly drunk anything."

No one was touching their food, and the steam rising from everyone's spaghetti was beginning to vanish.

"But imagine that one day that goblet fell and shattered into a thousand pieces."

"I get it," Ortal chimed in, her eyebrows arching, her head nodding. Maybe she did, at least in part.

I added that, despite the great disappointment over the goblet's loss, maybe we could see in the shattered glass a new kind of beauty.

"Sure, lots of little colored sparkles," Carmiel offered.

I asked how they could make something out of all those sparkles and not just sweep them into the trash.

"You could take the prettiest pieces," Carmiel continued, "and make a work of art out of them."

I agreed, offering that it could be some kind of mosaic.

Ortal responded, "So this is about you putting your life back together."

With a nod in her direction, I explained why I had wanted us to get together—so I could tell them about a new piece in my own mosaic. First, I reminded them of some of the pieces they already knew about: my work on the museum, my writing, my men's group, my regular workouts at the gym, and, of course, Jane.

"That's a lot of pieces," Jeremy offered.

I remarked that there was one more new piece.

I asked Jeremy, "Do you remember our little

dance in the park when I told you how much I was suffering from the burden of caring for Mom?"

He nodded.

"Well, actually, 'suffering' doesn't begin to express the feeling I've had now for some time. It's been more like—well, like I'm dying. Your mom, of course, is the one really dying, but I've been feeling like I am too, like everything around me is black and I seem unable to move, and the blackness will sweep over me and I'll be dead. But then, without my expecting it, life returned."

"I think I get it!" Ortal blurted out again. "Let me guess. Who is she?"

Faint smiles crept across the faces of Ariela and my grandchildren. Not Jeremy's face. Not Alon's.

I said that something very unexpected and unplanned had developed.

"Here comes the exciting part," Ishai declared, rolling his fork deep into his spaghetti and slurping up a mouthful.

"I have become close to someone," I said.

"I knew it!" Ortal exclaimed.

"How close?" Alon asked.

"Close."

"Who is she?" Jeremy asked.

"Who would you guess?" I asked.

They made a few wrong guesses. Then I took a deep breath, and on the exhale uttered, "Laura."

"Laura?" Carmiel burst out laughing. I had expected that from her. She had been in a relationship with Laura's eldest son in eleventh and twelfth grades. "If he and I were still together," Carmiel managed to squeak out, "we could go on a double date." Bowled over in laughter, she managed to add, "A three-generation double date!"

Ortal smiled broadly, as did Ishai, his teeth red with tomato sauce.

Ariela said, "Wow, Laura, she's a lot younger than you. How much?"

"Sixteen years," I answered.

"Go, go, go," Ishai's fist shot into the air, as though he were cheering a touchdown.

And then silence.

So far, I'd heard nothing from Jeremy or Alon. After a considerable pause, though, Jeremy spoke: "Dad, I'm happy for you. I'm thinking it's a good thing. But I'm also thinking, you know, about Mom, and it may take me some time to come to terms with this."

On my left, Alon was wagging his head from side to side. "So you're moving in with Laura?" he probed. "With Mom still alive?"

Everyone seemed to gag, including me.

"Of course not!" I reassured him that I would never leave his mom. I didn't add "the way your biological parents left you."

"I'm guessing that Mom knows about this," he said. "She must know, she's so smart."

"She *was* so smart," I answered, placing a hand on his. I told him that I was pretty sure she had no idea about it, but even if she suspected or wondered, she would probably forget it the next moment. What I didn't tell him was that I kept wondering whether her subconscious was still intact and whether, in some deep cognitive recess, she might sense Laura and me—or someone and me—but couldn't bring that intuition forth and express it.

I told Alon and Jeremy we could talk more about it whenever they wanted. While it was clear that Jeremy would need "some time to come to terms with it," it was also clear that Alon would need more than time and might never find peace with it.

| 21 |

Conditions in China

Not too bad, I noticed, turning sideways to my floor-to-ceiling bedroom mirror. Even without sucking in my stomach. Laura and I had been going to Weight Watchers for several months, though she came mostly to encourage me. I had recently increased my daily exercise regime and was creating a new relationship to food. "I don't need that" became my new mantra when high-calorie fare caught my eye. I had stopped eating bread, butter, cake, cookies, and ice cream—well, almost— and had developed a fondness for tomatoes, green peppers, cucumbers, and even the lowly mushroom. Within six months I had lost forty pounds. I stared again at the mirror, feeling pretty smug.

But what if, in spite of all this, the two-day bike tour Laura was planning as part of our imminent overseas trip were to prove too much for me? Laura was the cyclist, not me. What had I been thinking when I agreed to this tour? What was I trying to prove?

This would be our first trip overseas together. We were heading to the Far East, which, of course, reminded me of my time with Jane in Kyoto, a little over five years previously. Jane would never again be able to travel overseas, though I sensed that for Laura and me, this might be the first of many trips together.

But how would I tell Jane that I was going away for three weeks? Of course, I wouldn't mention Laura's participation. I had already told her about the first part of the trip, to Hong Kong, where I'd been invited to lecture at an international museum conference. She hadn't reacted, maybe because there was nothing new about my lecturing overseas. But how could I explain being away for three whole weeks? I'd considered pretending there was a second conference on mainland China. But she seemed oblivious to the whole discussion. My conscience eased somewhat when I confirmed the schedule of Jane's substantial team of visitors—the friends and family whose daily visits would continue while I was away. Armeda and Eunice would be with her full time as usual. Jeremy and Ariela would stay over a few nights each week. I told myself that Jane might not miss me at all. I wanted to believe that.

*   *   *

The upcoming trip seemed an appropriate occasion to conclude my sessions with Adina. I knew there was more I could learn from her, but at some point, I needed to take full responsibility for the complex life I was living, and, over the last year and a half, she had given me the tools for doing that. I was worried, though, that my quitting might insult her.

"I've been expecting your decision, and I think it's a good one" was Adina's reply.

I felt such admiration for her. I had so needed guidance, and she had truly come through for me.

*   *   *

A few weeks before the trip, I received an email from Jinhai, the tour guide for our cycling trip: "We bike sixty mile each day. South China coast very pretty. I hold place for you both?"

Did he say sixty? I had hardly ever cycled since my twenties, and even then, never sixty miles a day.

"They've got cars in China, don't they?" I chided Laura.

One morning at her place, we sat on the couch, sunlight pouring through a window onto a map spread across her lap. She traced out the planned bike route through China's southern Guangdong Province.

"We're going to love this ride," she said, "right between the shore and parklands at first and then climbing up into the hills."

"I've been thinking," I interjected. "Those sixty miles a day! I'm not so sure."

I reminded her that I had enjoyed our bike ride along the Tel Aviv boardwalk—that flat, straight, short boardwalk.

"Why do I sense I'm about to hear a 'but'?"

"Actually, you're about to hear a b-u-t-t."

I reminded her how, even on that short ride, the narrow, hard seat hurt my bony bottom. "Sixty miles of butt pain? I'm not so sure."

I suggested taking a step back and thinking it over again. I reminded her that I was open to new experiences, maybe even more than ever before, to which she nodded and said she loved me for that. But I also reminded her that I wasn't interested in a makeover.

"You're the cyclist here, not me." I suggested emailing Jinhai and requesting a different kind of tour. Less physical, more cultural.

"Okay," she replied, with a perceptible lack of enthusiasm.

In my next email to Jinhai, I stated my age, which he hadn't known.

He wrote back, "In your condition, we do thirty mile each day."

"In my what?" I shouted into thin air. Seventy-two was my age not my "condition!"

Nevertheless, I signed us up. "Thirty mile" it would be.

* * *

Three days after my Hong Kong lecture, Jinhai, a wiry, handsome, middle-aged man with a wispy black beard and a long black ponytail, showed up as scheduled at our hotel at 9:00 a.m. wearing jeans and a red T-shirt emblazoned with English writing: "Extreme cycle! Extreme fun!" His assistant, Ling, in her black biking outfit, looked to be in her late twenties.

They welcomed us into their minibus that already held eight other tourists.

Friendly greetings made the rounds, all in English but with French, German, and Scottish accents. A quick inspection revealed that I was by far the oldest member of the group. The youngest, an adorable girl about ten years old, wore a bright blue cycling jersey with a matching blue helmet and cycling gloves.

I took a seat between Laura and the ten-year-old for the one-hour drive to the bicycle rental shop and the start of our ride. Pulling off the glove on her right hand, our young companion reached out for a handshake. "Hello, Jeff, my name is Elizabeth," she said, in a sweet Scottish brogue, "and these are my parents." Smiles all around.

"Do you like bike riding, Elizabeth?" I asked.

"I love cycling! I go for a daylong ride almost every weekend with either my mom or my dad, way up into the mountains."

"Oh, good."

At the rental shop, Laura helped me pick out a suitable bike, and we fitted the padded seat cover we'd brought from Israel. That, together with my new padded bike shorts, should cushion me against pain.

The pace was easy as we set out along a mostly level, smoothly paved path. A white sandy beach on our left stretched some fifty yards from the path to gently breaking ocean waves. On our right, a bamboo forest was punctuated by kiosks selling coconuts, each cut open with a straw inserted. Many of the people walking on the path were sipping them, obviously a local favorite. We wove our way through walkers and other cyclists. Teen groups, adult singles, couples, and multigenerational families, almost all Chinese, appeared in good spirits, and I was happy to be sharing that spirit with them.

* * *

Despite my padded seat cover and shorts, I soon started to feel slight pain. Every few minutes, Laura asked me how I was doing, and I said fine, but I was a little less fine as time went on. Then, suddenly, the path's smooth surface changed to cobblestones. Within minutes, I was in serious pain. I tried sitting on the fleshier parts of my bottom, then on the top portion of either thigh, but these positions were awkward and largely unhelpful.

About five minutes later, I rode over to Jinhai and explained my predicament.

Jinhai kindly offered, "Take my bike; seat soft."

We exchanged bicycles, and after five minutes, he asked how I felt.

A little better, I told him, though the pain continued.

"Okay, restaurant for lunch just thirty minute from here. You can do?"

"Can do," I replied, unsure, however, whether I actually could do.

After half an hour of throbbing pain, we finally arrived at the outdoor restaurant on an isolated strip of beach. Elizabeth and her parents dashed to the sea and dipped their feet in the waves. Others strolled through the restaurant's beautiful garden or stepped into a shop selling a wide variety of seashells. I would have loved to look around inside but wasn't feeling up to it.

The hard truth hit me. I couldn't go on with the ride. I worried that if I told Jinhai, he might have to cancel or at least delay the rest of the day's ride, which would disappoint everyone, including Laura, of course. But I had no choice. I gave Jinhai the facts. Remarkably, without a moment's thought, he replied, "After lunch you,

Laura, me, we walk near here, very pretty." He said that Ling would cycle with the others, and we would all meet later at the hotel for dinner.

"Tomorrow, you two and me, we walk more."

This was clearly not Jinhai's first encounter with problem cyclists like me.

* * *

We all sat at a big, round table located outdoors on an elevated wooden platform. A slatted roof provided partial shade and a railing around the edge assured that none of us would fall off. The only non-Asians in the restaurant, our group stood out like a troop of foreign actors on a raised stage, with a sizable audience of diners seated at tables on the lawn below.

Jinhai and Ling said that this was considered the finest restaurant in Guangdong Province, and indeed the food lived up to that reputation. A delicious selection of fish, shellfish, vegetables, and rice with a variety of sauces were all beautifully presented in serving bowls placed on an enormous turntable centered on the dining table. By spinning it, each of us spooned out the several delectable items. But as I began to fill my plate, a sharp pain shot through my abdomen.

Nausea quickly ensued. The whole world began spinning around like that turntable. Leaning toward Laura, I whispered, "I'm going to faint."

And right there, in full view of all at our table, I slumped onto Laura's shoulder and passed out. I came to after about a minute, she told me later, as Jinhai was saying, "Hospital ten minute away. I call ambulance?"

From my stupor I called out, "No hospital, no ambulance," recalling the two occasions when I had fainted at the university during the past year. Each time I was rushed to the hospital by ambulance, sirens blaring, only to be sent home hours later. Both times, a sudden drop in blood pressure had caused my fainting, once when I had returned to work too soon following a bout of flu, and once after suffering an episode of intense pain resulting from gastric reflux. Nothing serious either time.

"Do you want to lie down on the floor?" Laura whispered.

She helped me onto my back and lifted my feet onto a chair, which made me feel better almost instantly. I closed my eyes in the warm comfort of the sun's rays filtering through the slatted roof.

"Listen, honey," she said, "I'm so sorry I got

you into this. When you said you weren't so sure about the cycling, I should have listened more closely."

"Laura, I need to rest. Why don't you go finish your lunch?"

My eyes still closed, I heard a chair pull up near me. Squinting in that direction, I was surprised to see a bright blue jersey.

"I'm very sorry you don't feel well, Jeff," Elizabeth consoled. "I'll take some photos of our cycling trip and I'll send them to you. Maybe sometime you can come to Scotland, and we can all walk together along some flat paths."

"That would be nice," I replied, managing half a smile. What a lovely child. I hoped we might have more of a conversation when I felt better.

I needed to get to the hotel and have some bed rest, and a taxi soon arrived to deliver Laura and me. Hopefully, the next day I would be up for the walking tour Jinhai had suggested.

And indeed, the next morning, I woke up feeling much better, and Jinhai guided us along a beautiful coastal path. During a break, as Jinhai headed off for coffee at a nearby kiosk, Laura and I relaxed on a bench overlooking the sea, refreshed by the moist breeze.

"Do you know what I was thinking yesterday, lying on that restaurant floor?" I asked.

"Let me guess. You wished you were back at the university?"

"No, I was fearing that you would see me as some old fart who can't do a simple bike ride, can't partner with you in what you love, and maybe can't partner with you at all, and maybe you're thinking you want out."

"Listen to me, Jeff. I admit I'm disappointed about the cycling. But be clear on one thing. I never wanted you because of your cycling skills."

"Well, that's good news!"

She added that cycling with her kids, her friends, organized groups, or alone, would fulfill her cycling urge. "So forget that. I want you!" she exclaimed.

We sat silently for a long time.

Jinhai returned and stood unobtrusively some distance away.

I reached for Laura's hand. We stood up and resumed our walk.

| 22 |

My Right to Life

I was surprised one day to receive an out-of-the-blue phone call from Adina. We hadn't spoken since our final session. She invited me to give a guest lecture to undergraduate students of occupational therapy in her course on aging. Specifically, she wanted the students to hear firsthand the personal struggle of an Alzheimer's caregiver. Struggle was certainly my story, and I was glad to share it.

Although I looked forward to being back in the classroom, I wondered whether the students would be able to bridge the vast span between their ages and mine; between their moving forward and upward and my efforts to escape the downward pull of both caring for Jane and my own aging. Would they feel free to express their thoughts—perhaps criticism—about certain things I might share with them?

About forty students filled the lecture hall, where bright sunlight streamed in through tall windows. After some introductory comments, I suggested, "Let's talk about love," which brought on many smiles.

"Love is a two-way street, wouldn't you agree?" I described love as something each partner both gives and receives in many different ways, but more or less in equal measure. It had been that way with Jane and me for nearly half a century, I explained.

"But now our love is like a one-way street—with me mostly giving and Jane receiving."

Sympathetic expressions reflected from several faces. It seemed that, yes, some of them, at least, did manage to cross the bridge to my elder self.

"Back-scratching, for instance," I continued, explaining that, whereas once Jane and I had each given and received, now it was only my hands on her back. I clarified that I love doing this, "but oooh, how I wish she could give me a good back scratch like she used to!" With this, I rolled my shoulders, swiveled on my hips, and squeezed my eyes shut. Laughter filled the room. But softly, compassionately. I even spied a few students dabbing their eyes.

Changing direction, I continued. "Let me tell you how I started learning some hard lessons about things I could do for myself to help relieve the heaviness and sadness as Jane's Alzheimer's deepened."

I felt so uncomfortable, I told them, the first time I bought just one ticket to a concert, but how thrilling it had been to hear Yuja Wang at the keyboard. Then I described a few of Adina's suggestions that had sounded so unrealistic when she'd first broached them. Going away alone overnight to a hotel, for instance. Impossible. Who would care for Jane? But I explained how Adina had advised me to arrange visits to Jane by family and friends while I was away, and afterward she helped me set up regular once-a-week visits, each a few hours long, by several of those family and friends—what a breakthrough. And full-time hired helpers? No thanks; at first I didn't want strangers living in the house. Yet, ultimately, hiring Armeda and Eunice greatly eased my burden and brought a measure of joy back into our lives. And with their presence, together with the visits of family and friends, I managed to have time for my own work activities, and even for overseas travel.

I felt the students were with me. But I had not yet told them about Laura, and I worried how they might respond. But I reminded myself, these students are professionals-in-training; they need to deal with this.

* * *

"I'd like to share with you one more change I've made that may surprise you. It certainly surprised me. And some of you may find it a bit shocking."

I took a deep breath, exhaled, and then gradually introduced the subject. I explained the early meetings with Laura to discuss, initially, our writing and the family challenges we were each facing. What I hadn't expected, I told them, was that these discussions would draw Laura and me closer together.

It became personal.

It became intimate.

It became love.

Secret love, of course.

"Yes, at seventy-two, I've fallen deeply in love. With a woman sixteen years my junior. And she returns that love."

There were whispers.

Downcast eyes.

Slinking in chairs.

I clarified that my love for Jane had not waned one bit and I was certain it never would. I repeated, however, that this love was mostly unidirectional and limited by her incapacity.

A student in the front row raised her hand, shaking her head back and forth, her long curly hair flopping from side to side. She blurted out, "This doesn't sit well with me. Jane didn't choose to be sick. You're still married to her, right? Yet you're in love with someone else?"

I took a deep breath and then began by thanking her for her openness.

I said I'd like to respond primarily to her question about my still being married. "When your spouse has become no longer like a spouse but more like a child, even a very young child in diapers, when she is unable to feed herself or to care for her own bodily needs, when her speech is reduced to a few words so there can be no chatting about the kids and grandkids or about what you did that day, or what to have for dinner, when the two of you sleep in different bedrooms—hers with one of the caregivers; then as much as you may still love her—and I do and always will—to what extent is there still a marriage?"

She leaned back in her chair, still shaking her head.

"What's he supposed to do?" a young man sitting toward the back of the room called out. "He has no choice."

"He certainly does have a choice," she shot back, glaring at him over her shoulder, "to stick with his wife and her only."

Murmuring spread throughout the class. I sensed that most of them sided with the front-row student. One of them called out to her, "I'm with you. He married Jane, and that's supposed to be a lifelong commitment. And now he's leaving her just because she's sick?"

"Hold on," I interrupted, "who said anything about leaving? Jane and I live together in our home with me loving her."

"Okay, but at some point, you'll move her to a nursing home so you can be with your new woman, right?"

"Of course not! Why would you think that? Jane is with me in our home to the end. I've never even imagined her being anywhere else."

I shifted direction and reiterated that the various things I'd been doing for myself—from buying that single concert ticket to pursuing my relationship with Laura—were very important to me. I didn't view any of them as flip decisions. "Why do you think these things are so important to me?" I asked the students.

The agitated front row student answered, "I think it's all about how they can make you a better caregiver for Jane. If you were depressed or something, how could you help her?"

Another student commented, "Yes, but also it's just good for you, regardless of Jane."

I agreed with both, but said I'd like to follow up on what the second student had said: "Let me rephrase your comment. You might have said that I have a right to life." I looked around the room, trying to catch as many eyes as possible. "Just like you," I said, pointing to one of them, "and you," pointing to another, and then another. "Just like each of you, I have a right to life. That right doesn't cease to exist when you become old like me."

I explained that I needed to repeat these thoughts to myself often because it was a hard lesson for me to learn. There was no need for me to stop living because of Jane's Alzheimer's. "If I did that, there would be two deaths, so to speak, not just one."

I added that, thanks to the things I've learned to do for myself, I've been able to grow in many new directions. And though deeply sad about Jane, all those new directions I was allowing myself, including my connection with Laura, made me feel alive and grateful for life.

A student sitting by the windows half raised her hand, as if unsure whether she wanted to speak. I nodded to her.

"Do you feel guilty?" she asked, almost in a whisper.

That question threw me. At first I didn't know how to answer. To give myself a few moments of thought, I asked the student, "Do *you* think I'm guilty?"

"I can't say," she replied. "I've never been where you are, married for nearly a lifetime, and now Jane's illness."

Looking directly at her, I replied, "Yes, I feel guilty." I paused to let that sink in—both for her and for myself. "But guilt is only half of what I feel. The other half is what I said earlier—that I have a right to life." I paused to gather my thoughts. "What's needed is to find the balance between these two seeming opposites." With the word "balance," I turned my hands palms up and moved them up and down in alternation like the pans on a scale of justice.

I checked my watch. With just a few minutes left, I told the class that I wanted to leave them with a challenge.

"I'm guessing that some of you will become professionals dealing with the elderly, and you may have occasion to advise people like me who are caring for someone with Alzheimer's or another form of dementia. Some of these caregivers may choose to act in ways that you will find objectionable." I clarified that I was not speaking of actions that would endanger anyone or break any laws. "If and when this happens, here's my challenge: set aside your own personal feelings and moral judgments. Encourage that caregiver's choice, even if you disagree with it."

"That caregiver has a right to life.

"That caregiver needs your help.

"So help that person.

"Save a life."

| 23 |

The Hook

The morning after my lecture, I sat up in bed thinking about some of the comments that Adina's students had made. One was the assumption that I would move Jane into a nursing home. I had replied no, Jane was with me to the end. Yet, there I was in our bedroom, without Jane. I had moved her not to a nursing home, of course, but to the downstairs bedroom, and for her own protection against falling. Since her move, I would sometimes half wake in the night, reach over to feel where she used to be, only to face the reality that her Alzheimer's had already swept her away from me, if only to the downstairs.

Sitting up in bed now, I looked around the room at the various signs of Jane, particularly the reminders of her intellectual and creative life. The journals she'd written on and off, from high school until she could no longer write, filled three shelves above her computer. The corner bookcase displayed several identical books titled *Women Against Women*, the published version of Jane's PhD thesis in which she had analyzed the American women who had opposed women's right to vote in the 1920s. Jane had dedicated the book: "To my mother, born in America before women could vote, and to my two granddaughters, growing up in the young country where I now live, a country that has already seen one woman prime minister." On the wall hung a framed but faded poster advertising the play "Mrs. Satan," about Victoria Woodhull, the first woman to run for US president, which Jane had written in collaboration with a drama professor. Its college performance had earned very positive reviews.

* * *

There was another place, though, that touched me even more deeply than Jane's displayed accomplishments. I stood up from bed and stepped into the spacious walk-in closet that now held just my clothes, Jane's having been moved to her downstairs bedroom. Two shiny, metal hooks protruded from the closet's back wall. There, on most mornings, Jane and I would slip out of our pajamas, hang them on those hooks, and usually give each other a hug or a kiss before taking the day's clothes from the shelves. The hook on the left had always been mine, the other, Jane's. But ever since her move downstairs, I had kept her hook empty. I sensed that hanging my own clothes on it would snuff out my memory of those blissful morning moments. But more, I sensed that hook was still Jane's.

On this day, as I left the closet, a chilling November breeze wafted in through the bedroom window—time for me to start changing over to my winter nightwear. So once I'd dressed, I pulled out a pair of my flannel pajamas from our bedroom's off-season clothes cabinet and carried them back into the walk-in closet. There I stood before those two hooks, mine draped with the summer pajamas that I would still need on the odd warm night, and Jane's hook empty. Would I betray the tender memory of Jane hanging her pajamas by appropriating her hook?

A voice inside me proclaimed, "It's just a hook." Hesitantly, I draped my winter garments there.

Once dressed and walking downstairs, I came to a stark realization—Jane and her PJs being gone from the closet was a prelude to, ultimately, Jane being gone.

PART IV

LANDING

| 24 |

Hard to Swallow

On a cold, rainy January morning, about six and a half years since Kyoto, I awoke with worries buzzing through my brain. Jane had developed a problem with swallowing food or pills. Dr. Ban had prescribed particular pills that I had bought the previous evening, and she was to take the first one this morning after breakfast. But they were large pills, and I worried whether she could swallow them.

Dr. Ban had explained to me the complications with Jane's swallowing. Getting food (or pills) from the mouth to the throat involves several acts that, he said, are so simple that they seem automatic, but they actually require cognitive decisions. Like deciding to close and tighten the lips, to move the tongue so as to position the food first for chewing and then for swallowing, and finally to initiate the actual gulp which, once begun, proceeds automatically. Most people don't consciously think about those decisions, he clarified, but for someone with Alzheimer's, even such seemingly simple matters can present a challenge.

* * *

I went downstairs and settled onto the couch alongside the sleeping Golani. Lately, he had deserted his little bed on the floor for the corner of the couch beside where Jane most frequently sat.

Soon Armeda began her morning singsong: "Waking time, Jane, I get you up now."

She kept up the chant, as she did every morning, while removing Jane's pajamas and diaper, cleaning her, and lifting her onto the wheelchair. Jane had become so thin that Armeda was able to do all this with relative ease.

"OK, we make shower now, you like that," she chirped, wheeling Jane from bedroom to bathroom.

I heard the water running and then, suddenly, Jane screaming, "Hot! Hot! Out! Out!"

Those were the most words I'd heard from her in the past few days.

"Sorry, Jane dear, better now?"

A few minutes later, "I get you dry now and brush your teeth. Then we have breakfast with Jeff." Eunice was already clanking pots and dishes in the kitchen.

We assembled at the table, Jane wearing fresh pajamas and a bathrobe with pictures of dogs. I kissed her damp, curly, white hair and inhaled its lemony-shampoo scent. Running my hand down her back brought forth her faint smile. With each upward scratching stroke, she leaned forward and lowered her head. With each sideways stroke, she swiveled according to my movements.

Eunice brought in my oatmeal and Jane's soft-boiled egg. Armeda lifted a half-filled teaspoon. But Jane clamped her lips shut. Wrinkles like rain gutters furrowed her face from the corners of her eyes and down her cheeks.

"You open now, Jane," Armeda said patiently three times, and the third time Jane did open.

Armeda tilted the spoon upward and the egg spilled onto Jane's tongue. She didn't swallow at first, and some of the egg dribbled out one corner of her mouth—just as Dr. Ban had explained, a failed decision about swallowing. Finally, she did gulp the egg down, with her eyes shut tight and her face scrunched up.

After swallowing a few teaspoons of egg, she refused to take in any more. It was time for her orange pill, which nearly half-filled a teaspoon. Armeda pressed the spoon against Jane's lower lip while Eunice stood by with a glass of water.

This isn't going to work, I thought to myself.

"Okay, now you take pill," Armeda said.

But Jane didn't take it into her mouth. Rather, she clasped it between her lips and held it, half in her mouth and half out, like an acorn protruding from a bird's beak.

"Okay, now drink," Eunice said, raising a glass of water, but as the glass approached Jane's lips, the pill disappeared into her mouth. She wrinkled her nose, wagged her head violently from side to side, and raised both hands as if to protect herself from an onslaught. Armeda grabbed Jane's chin to steady her as Eunice inserted the rim of the glass between Jane's lips and tilted it, but most of the water flowed straight down Jane's chin and onto Armeda's hand and arm. Jane started coughing violently. Between coughing spells, she opened her eyes wide, shook her head, and seemed unable to take in air.

"Where is pill?" Armeda cried out.

Fear projected from Jane's wide-open eyes.

I patted her back lightly, then harder, but she kept on coughing and couldn't catch her breath.

I grabbed my cell phone and dialed 101 for an ambulance.

"My wife is choking!" I shouted to the dispatcher.

Is she conscious? Yes. How is her breathing? Only occasional, between coughs, with heavy wheezing. What color is her skin? Whitish.

Within minutes an intensive-care team arrived by motorcycle. The medics connected Jane to oxygen, which eased her breathing, and her coughs soon decreased to brief bouts. The pill was nowhere to be seen, probably swallowed somehow.

Then the ambulance arrived, and the team lifted Jane onto a stretcher, a blanket wrapped around her, and carried her out to the street, accompanied by Armeda, Eunice, and me. A stiff wind whipped a cold drizzle across our faces. They rolled Jane into the ambulance, with Armeda, Eunice, and one team member climbing in next to her, and the driver pulled away.

I would drive myself to the hospital soon.

But I couldn't get myself to hurry.

I knew that the intake procedure would be lengthy, and that Jane was in good hands.

I needed to return to the place Jane had last occupied in our house, the dining table. I needed to make order there.

I cleared and washed the dishes. Wiped the table and the kitchen counters. Straightened the chairs.

I stood still there for some time, sensing the silence. This was the first time in a long while that I had been alone in the house, even for just moments, and I didn't like it.

I drove to the hospital.

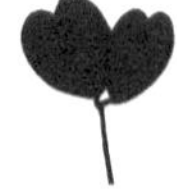

| 25 |

No More

“I’ll kill you!” Jane shrieked at me when I arrived at her bedside in the emergency ward, her face contorted, her gnarled fingers digging into my arm.

Ten minutes later I returned from the coffee machine. “I love you,” she whispered, her face smooth, her hands relaxed.

She said nothing else to me that day.

A middle-aged doctor entered, read Jane’s medical chart, asked who I was, and told me that the recommended treatment in Jane’s condition was what he called a PEG—a feeding tube, he clarified. Installed under general anesthesia, the tube would extend from outside Jane’s abdomenal skin directly to her stomach, and she would take all her food and liquid by this route. There would be no more swallowing problems.

I must have looked incredulous.

"We do this procedure all the time," he said.

"Not this time," I told myself, on Jane's behalf. If the anesthesia didn't kill her, the indignation would.

"She'll pull out the tube," I told the doctor.

"We can tie her hands."

"You can *what?*"

* * *

Jane developed pneumonia in the hospital. She stayed there for over a week, receiving infusions of antibiotics but growing perceptably weaker by the day.

When we finally brought her home, she mostly sat slumped in her wheelchair, her head hanging, like a worn-out rag doll.

One day, she refused to get out of bed and never did again.

I woke early one morning, dressed, and went downstairs. To my surprise, Jane was already awake, covered by a blue quilt, her head propped up on two pillows. Armeda and Eunice were in the kitchen.

I sat on the edge of her bed, holding her hand, and she gazed up at me.

"Good morning, my dear," I chatted. "I have a question for you. Do you remember when we first met? In the hallway outside my Cambridge apartment? And how you climbed in through my window? And pulled me out of bed so we could exercise? Do you remember?"

"Yes," she whispered.

"And then we got really friendly. Remember?"

No answer, just a smile.

"And then we got married, not just once like most couples. Three times. Chinese gong and all."

A faint smile.

"Love each other for what you are ..."

I choked on these words and couldn't complete the phrase.

Her eyes remained closed now, and she gave no response. Her blue quilt continued to rise and fall with each breath.

Pressing my lips to her forehead, I knew what I had always known—I still loved her after half a century, even across the great divide to wherever her aging brain, her brain disorder, her brain degeneration, and finally her Alzheimer's had taken her.

* * *

One night Alon came over to see Jane. I sat on the edge of her bed while he, of course, sat in his wheelchair. From his first year until his twentieth, this had been his room, his bed. It pained me to see him there, viewing his mother that way.

I recalled the first time I'd ever seen him, Jane holding him in her arms as I worked my way slowly toward them along the hallway of the disabled children's hospital.

"She found you," I whispered to Alon.

The reservoir of tears he had stored up until that moment suddenly burst forth.

"She *saved* me," he squeaked, tears spilling down his cheeks.

I bent down and kissed his forehead, and he reached his arms up and around my neck, as he had that moment when Jane first handed him to me, and I first felt the electric energy in his grasp. And now we watched together as his mother's energy slowly faded from her life.

* * *

Within a few days, Jane stopped eating altogether and barely drank. One night, just before she fell asleep, I sat on the edge of her bed and looked into her half-open eyes. We were alone.

"I love you," I whispered, not knowing whether she could hear me. But with great effort, she leaned her head ever-so-slightly forward, and I leaned down, kissed her lips, and felt her kiss me back. Then again. Five times in all I kissed her, and five times she returned my kisses.

Alone with her again the next night, I sat on her bed and again I said, "I love you." Again she leaned forward, but this time she returned just two of my five kisses. Something in me said these were the last two kisses she would ever give me, and I vowed never to forget them.

On a still later night, her face was expressionless, cheeks emaciated, eyes sunken, her lips open in the shape of an *O*. As I held her hand, her eyes turned toward me, but her head didn't move. Dr. Ban came by after his workday. Jane had barely woken up over the past two days. After examining her, he turned to me. "I'm so sorry, Jeff, but I think that Jane might take her last breath some time before morning."

* * *

For six and a half years, ever since Kyoto, Jane had been losing more and more of herself. Now she hardly had anything more to lose.

Jeremy and Ariela stayed over with me, and we divided the night watch between us. Ariela took the first shift and agreed to wake me at 1:00 a.m.

But when I opened my eyes, the sun was already up. What was going on? Had Ariela fallen asleep and therefore not woken me? I threw on a bathrobe and headed downstairs.

On the living room couch, Jeremy and Golani were both half asleep. Ariela was awake and sitting next to Jane's bed. She had decided to stay up all night and let me sleep. To my surprise, Jane was still breathing, though weakly.

Ariela whispered, "She waited for you."

Those soft words pierced my heart. Really? Could she possibly have done that? Did she somehow sense that, after spending most of our lives together, she couldn't depart without saying to me, in some silent language, goodbye?

I sat on the edge of her bed and held her hand. Within moments her breaths became even more shallow.

Jeremy walked in and sat at the foot of the bed.

Few breaths now, separated by pauses.

A single breath. A pause.
Another breath. A very long pause.
Another.
Then no more.

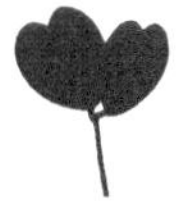

| 26 |

Shiva

The simple cloth shroud revealed the contours of Jane's body as they carried her on a stretcher at sundown, past many gravestones, to her own space, dug out waiting to receive her. They lowered her, carefully positioning her shrouded body, then erected around and over her a casing of cinder blocks.

Someone handed me a shovel. At first it just dangled from my hand. After some moments, I scooped it half full of pebbly soil and tilted it over the grave. The falling pebbles pounded the cinder block casing. Then silence.

Others followed after me, shoveling earth up to the grave's brim. At that moment, I understood what is widely known about the Jewish tradition of shoveling: only when you, your family, and your friends have covered your loved one with earth—only then do you know, deep down, that it's over.

As darkness set in, I went back home with Jeremy and his family, Alon and his helper Priyantha, Armeda, and Eunice. It had all happened so fast. Just ten hours earlier, Jane had taken her last breath; just three hours earlier, she had lain shrouded during the eulogies; two hours earlier, I had walked behind the stretcher to her grave, and then the shoveling.

Now, sitting on the living room couch among my children and grandchildren, without Jane, I wept uncontrollably.

"I left her behind!

"In the dirt!

"I just walked away and left her there!"

* * *

I woke early the next morning, somewhat dreading the day's events, the beginning of the seven days of Shiva, the most intense period of mourning. I didn't feel like greeting visitors; I didn't want to be "on."

More than anything, I wanted to take a long walk, alone, in the woods. I wanted to find a place, not there in the woods, but inside myself. A place where I might be able to connect with Jane, speak to her, ask her questions, and imagine her answers. But I had no idea how to do that or if it was even possible.

Following the traditional morning prayer service, the house began to fill up. I hadn't expected so many people.

I soon realized there was no need for me to be "on." No social demands were made, and I appreciated people coming. Some visitors said little. A few uttered traditional Jewish expressions such as, "May God comfort you among the other mourners of Zion." Others shared memories of Jane, of me, or of our whole family.

Pleasant as everyone's comments were, they did little to ease my mind. The place within me where I might connect with Jane still eluded me.

* * *

Ken, a man in his fifties, sat down beside me on the couch. He had immigrated to Israel from America at about the same time as Jane and me. He and Jane met as Pardes students and, in spite of their age difference, became close friends.

Ken spoke to me in a manner that was different from everyone else. He asked me several probing questions, like, "What was it like for you as Jane approached her end?" To answer,

I shared one of our last moments of intimacy: "She leaned slightly forward in her bed. It was very hard for her. We kissed twice and then never again."

Now I wondered what Jane had felt at the moment of our two kisses.

Was she kissing me goodbye?

Did she feel sadness?

Did she feel at peace?

Did she feel love?

My questions for Jane just kept flowing.

I then realized that my discussion with Ken had led me to the very place within myself that I had been seeking.

It had been a long while since I had asked Jane questions like these; now that she was gone, I could do that again.

PART V

AFTER

| 27 |

Bargello

Shabbat morning, the first day after the Shiva, six thirty on my bedside clock, and the first light from a wintry sky filtered in through the curtains.

Armeda and Eunice were gone, having moved out the day before.

All the visits were over.

Finally, alone.

It was what I wanted. I'd even declined two lunch invitations.

But what was I going to do alone in my house all day?

I pulled the blankets over me and shut my eyes. But no luck. Seven o'clock. Seven thirty. I slipped into my robe and slippers and started padding down the stairs.

With the living room in view, I suddenly recalled that I was not totally alone. There lay

Golani, near Jane's favorite place on the couch, raising his head with a yawn and a soft groan.

I sat and petted him on his long, floppy ears, just as Jane often had.

That gave me an idea—touching some other things that Jane had often touched might help me feel in contact with her.

I went into her room, sat at her desk, and rummaged through its deep bottom drawer. I came up with her car keys. Closing my fingers over them, I recalled something she had admitted to me after she'd stopped driving. Several times, when I had walked into town or was buried in my writing upstairs, she had gone out to the car, sat in the driver's seat, started the engine, and shifted into first, then reverse, then first again, each time rolling just a few feet forward or back. Though confined within the three painted white lines of our disabled parking space, she wished herself out on a highway—the once freewheeling Kerouac devotee, now imprisoned within three white lines.

On the bookshelf above Jane's desk stood a heavy volume I hadn't noticed in years: *ASCAP Biographical Dictionary, Fourth Edition*. It was her father's book that she had kept all those years: a collection of brief biographical sketches of more than two thousand American songwriters and lyricists with lists of their compositions.

I found Jane's dad on page 252. Among the listed compositions was the one that Jane had mentioned to me some fifty years earlier at our first shared dinner and that I had played for Jerome when I met him in their New York apartment—"Love Is Like a Cigarette."

I walked into the living room and searched on the shelves for the file Jane had kept of her father's sheet music. There, beside my *Broadway Hits of the Sixties* and *The Just Jazz Real Book* was a manila folder stuffed with pages of his lyrical output. I pulled out the sheet music for "Love Is Like a Cigarette."

As my fingers swept across the keyboard, I glanced sideways and imagined Jane sitting there in her wheelchair listening. It was the type of musical moment we had often shared during her illness. There was just enough space for her wheelchair between the piano and the closet behind her.

When I finished the song, I looked again, and she was gone. All I saw was the closet door. Not having opened that door for as long as I could remember, I walked over, looked inside, and found decades of forgotten items: old camping equipment recalling our early trips to New Hampshire's White Mountains and the Adirondacks, two folded beach chairs we would sometimes take with us to Tel Aviv, and several boxes stuffed with papers and old magazines.

One box was curiously labeled "Bargello" in Jane's handwriting. I pried open the flaps and there discovered an exquisite wool needlepoint in a geometric pattern of dark brown, russet, beige, and cream. Of course! Back in our Ithaca days, Jane had taken up Bargello needlepoint. This piece had probably not been seen for thirty years.

I sat back down on the piano bench and spread the fabric across my lap. I turned it upside down, and so many threads poked up at me, like a thousand tiny fingers, each individually stitched in place. I had wanted to touch things of Jane's, and this felt almost like touching her fingers many times over. I wondered if it might fit on the piano bench, replacing its badly worn upholstered cover. Maybe that was what Jane had planned when she wove it.

I stood up and draped the needlepoint over the bench. Almost but not quite; it was just a bit too small. Disappointed, I folded it back into its box and put it back in the closet.

I later recalled that Jeremy worked with a very good upholsterer, whom I looked up. After discussing the matter with him, I invited him to add a modest off-white surround to frame Jane's beautiful multicolored Bargello, making a lovely bench cover.

What a wonderful, unexpected gift from Jane.

From then on, each time I sat at the piano, I would sense Jane's thousand little wool "fingers" massaging me right where I sat.

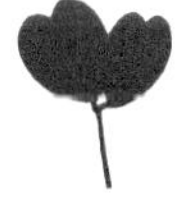

| 28 |

Signs

By a few months after Jane's death, I felt able to think back quite clearly over the six and a half years of her illness. Painfully, I realized that I had little awareness of what Jane really knew and felt about herself throughout that time. We had hardly ever talked about it, which must have made it worse for her, as it surely did for me.

One of the things that lifted my spirits somewhat was that photo on my piano of Jane standing strong and seemingly healthy on that Annapurna ledge, taken several years before Kyoto.

But one thing puzzled me about her trek up that mountain. Shortly after she came back, Jane told me that my decision not to join her on that trip had ultimately been a good thing, as it made the trip more her own. I'd never asked what she meant by that.

I was delighted, therefore, when Naomi, Jane's Annapurna trekking partner, phoned me one Friday morning and said she had a question for me and would like to drop in for a chat.

I made coffee for two and moved Jane's Annapurna photo to the dining room table.

* * *

Naomi arrived bearing one of her signature carrot cakes.

"Ah, my favorite picture," she exclaimed, glancing at the table. "I'm proud to have snapped that one."

We sat over cake and coffee and talked about their Annapurna trip.

"Do you have any idea what Jane meant," I asked, "when she said that Annapurna was more her own trip because I wasn't with her?"

She clanked her cup down on the saucer, then picked it up again, but didn't sip, and clanked it down again. She drew in a deep breath before saying, "I've been trying to remember when Jane started … you know … drifting away." With those words, she waved her hand over the photograph as if Jane were drifting right off the mountain.

I repeated what I had told her previously: it first happened in Kyoto when Jane had become strangely confused at a T-junction.

Naomi's eyes darted about for a moment as if searching for her next thought.

"Actually, I was wondering if it might have begun earlier than that," she said. "Maybe even a good deal earlier."

She lifted the photo and stared at it. "I first noticed something right here on this mountain. Most mornings, when we started our trekking, Jane couldn't figure out whether we were supposed to walk uphill or down. She needed me or our guide to point the way."

I bolted back in my chair. "Naomi, are you sure? That was more than twelve years ago!"

"Yes, and one more thing," she murmured. "Most nights we slept in a shelter with no indoor plumbing. If Jane needed to go to the outhouse, she usually couldn't find it. Or she couldn't find her way back. I was afraid she'd get lost during the night, maybe even fall right off the mountain. So I told her to wake me, and I always made sure to go there and back with Jane, holding her hand."

Once again, a problem with direction, I agonized.

Naomi's revelation triggered an earlier memory about Jane and direction. We would often take a twenty-minute walk from our house in downtown Jerusalem to certain shops on Jaffa Road. As we left the house, Jane always wanted to turn right, though the route was clearly shorter and no less pleasant if we turned left. I explained, cajoled, and even pointed out the route on a map. But nothing helped. She would just give a nonchalant backward wave of her hand, saying, "Yes, but it's this way," and turn right. This disagreement went on for decades. Finally, I gave in and simply turned right, sometimes even when Jane wasn't with me. Just a Jane idiosyncrasy, I'd always thought. I wouldn't have given it another thought if Naomi and I were not having our conversation.

"Jeff, I never wanted to mention these things before." Naomi said. "You had enough going on. But there is one more thing, if you're interested."

I nodded.

"Jane carried a very small backpack, while the guide and I both carried bigger ones. Every morning Jane would unpack and repack it. Then unpack and repack again, and again, even though there was very little in it. If I hadn't helped her, we'd never have gotten out onto the trail."

That reminded me of Jane's packing for trips from way back, probably even from back in Ithaca—over thirty years ago! Packing had always confounded Jane. Whenever we went away for a few weeks or just overnight, she would pack and repack time and again, just as Naomi described. I'd always put it down to simple indecision.

I didn't know whether these small confusions from way back were early signs of a developing cognitive problem or just ordinary idiosyncrasies. Not that it mattered now, but I was curious.

Naomi glanced at her watch, and I knew she had to leave. Though we both stood up, neither of us turned toward the door.

"But I still don't understand why Jane needed me to be absent from Annapurna in order to feel the trip was her own."

Naomi paused, clearing her throat a few times, then, "There's something she asked me not to tell you." She paused again. "But now, well, I guess nothing can hurt her."

I kept silent, hoping she would go on.

"One day when we were up on the mountain, Jane said, 'Please don't tell Jeff about the packing and unpacking, about my sense of direction, and all … you know, about my brain.'"

I fell into the nearest chair.

She knew!

Way back then, more than twelve years ago, she already knew!

I breathed deeply and tried to collect my thoughts. It wasn't clear what exactly she knew, but she obviously sensed that her mind was not all there.

Now I could see why she felt that with me present, it wouldn't have been her trip. I'd have noticed her problems and felt a need to take care of her, make decisions, take charge, maybe even end the trip early and get back to Israel to see a doctor.

After Naomi left, I couldn't stop thinking about Jane keeping it all secret and how we had never spoken openly about her illness.

Maybe if Jane had talked to me about her fears, we could have explored what it was like for us both. We might have found whole new ways of coming together while she was still able to converse.

But no, I couldn't blame Jane for our silence; I was at least as much to blame. That's how I was, how I'd grown up.

I was left saddened that the Jane in the photo was already not the Jane she had been, who had previously climbed so many mountains, climbed through my Cambridge window, climbed academically up through a PhD, and "climbed" to Israel. (Immigrating to Israel is referred to in Hebrew as aliya, which means ascent.) And, yet, from what Naomi told me, the Jane of that photo must have known that Annapurna would be her final ascent.

| 29 |

Fashion

I was happy to be going to Jeremy and Ariela's house for dinner. It was early spring, and it would be my first time there since I'd informed them that Laura and I were a couple. This time I came without a mission.

My granddaughter Carmiel greeted me at the front door. She leaned back and took a long look at me. "Something's wrong with your pants," she asserted. "Too baggy." She kept looking. "Your shirt too." She was twenty-four and, as she would put it, "into fashion."

I slipped past her, muttering, "They're comfortable."

"But you've lost all that weight," Carmiel replied, following me, "with your dieting and exercise."

"Not dieting," I protested over my shoulder, "my new relationship to food."

"Okay, but along with all your not dieting, you should buy some new clothes."

Ariela, hearing the conversation, looked me over and nodded agreement with her daughter.

All this surprised me. They knew I was a casual dresser, and they'd never commented before. I liked loosely fitting clothes. They allowed for air circulation. True, my pants and shirt were a bit floppy on me, but was that really a problem?

Back at home that night, I faced the full-length mirror in my bedroom. I saw what Carmiel had meant, though I still wondered why all the attention to my pants and shirts. They're only clothes. What really matters, I told myself, is who's wearing them.

* * *

The next morning, bearing a load of freshly washed laundry to the terrace clothesline, I clipped three pairs of white underpants onto the line with a single clothespin. They hung there, slightly slumped against one another. Next came three white T-shirts, also slumped together and singly pinned. I hung the remaining items in pairs. Within five minutes, the laundry basket was empty.

This was very different from what had been Jane's laundry care on our terrace. She would spread out each item, hang it separately using two clips, and then smooth the fabric between her palms, almost lovingly. For her, hanging laundry was also part of a wider ritual. She'd scan the flowers and trees she'd planted around the terrace perimeter, pulling a weed here, pruning a branch there. She would take in the panoramic view of the nearby park, the Knesset, and the Supreme Court. Sometimes she would sit either alone or with a friend in our rickety old terrace chairs. The terrace seemed to be her favorite place in the house.

But for me, it was different. Get the clothes on and off the line with minimal labor and maximum speed and then move on. Who cares how the clothes dry? They're only clothes.

I did notice, however, that some of my underpants and T-shirts were looking threadbare. This, together with their being rather big on the new me, made me think that sometime soon I might need to invest in new underwear.

* * *

On a subsequent trip to New York, I visited Macy's, where I searched for and found Jockey, my underwear brand. And there before me was something I'd never before set eyes on—stacks and stacks of black underpants and T-shirts. Black! All my life I'd known that men's underwear was white. True, women had been more experimental in this regard (so I'd been told). But men? My scant interest in fashion suddenly challenged, I boldly loaded up on pitch-black undergarments.

Back in Jerusalem, I paraded about Laura's bedroom one morning in my new black underwear.

"Why, Professor Camhi, what's that you've got on?" she asked. "It looks *very* attractive!"

Such a comment, from such a person, can change your whole outlook on fashion.

The next morning, Laura looked on as I donned a beige sport shirt over a black T-shirt. I left the top button open, of course, which left my new undershirt's neckline barely visible, like a baby blackbird peeking over the edge of the nest.

Laura gave that a look, then reached up and unbuttoned my next-to-top button. "That's more like it," she said, "two open buttons."

I looked in the mirror. "Radical!" I muttered. And from that moment on, I became a committed two-button radical.

* * *

Despite my foray into undergarments and buttons, I held firm in my stance that what really matters is not what's on the body but what's in the mind and the heart.

Eventually, though, that viewpoint conflicted with another, namely, that my clothes, like my facial expression and body posture, express how I feel about myself and how I would like others to regard me. While obvious to some, for me this was new terrain.

In due course, I went on to make a clean break from my oversized trousers. With Laura by my side, I visited a department store in a Jerusalem mall. There I skidded past the slim-fit pants racks, realizing that were I to wear those items, my legs would look and feel like salamis stuffed into a taut skin. I envisioned the words *Hebrew National* running down my thigh.

I asked a saleslady, "Do you have anything a bit less slim fit?" She pointed to the far corner of the store. The very far corner. There we found a few nice-looking pants that fit me well. Trying them on felt like stepping into a new persona. Laura helped me pick out some new shirts and sweaters as well.

I left the mall feeling ever so slightly a new man.

Ever so slightly into fashion.

| 30 |

Jane's Place

inner for two was warming in the kitchen when Laura arrived on a mid-summer evening. She looked lovely in a floral dress that I hadn't seen before. She smiled, noting my new pants and the two open buttons of my new shirt. She probably expected we'd be eating in the dining room, as we had several times during the six months since Jane's death. As I greeted her with a hug, she looked over my shoulder at the empty table and asked whether I'd like her to set it.

"No need," I replied, loading serving dishes onto two trays. I asked her to take one and follow me. We walked through the living room, past the couch where Golani looked up and sniffed, past the piano where Jane looked out at us from her Annapurna photo, and over to the stairway where Laura flashed me a suspicious smile.

As I mounted the first step, I hesitated. I had selected for our dinner the terrace off our bedroom. But the terrace had been Jane's favorite place. Was this a wise choice?

Upstairs, we walked through the bedroom and out onto the terrace.

"My goodness!" Laura exclaimed, clearly impressed by the new look. I had removed the clotheslines and stored Jane's collection of gardening tools behind the potted cypress trees. The two rickety old chairs were gone, replaced by two new padded metal armchairs and a matching round table that I had set elegantly for dinner with candles burning inside glass wind protectors. Also new were two chaise lounges, each made up with a pillow and a light blanket. On a separate serving table I had placed an open bottle of Cabernet Sauvignon, two wine glasses, assorted appetizers, and two chafing dishes to keep our dinner warm until served.

"It was always so lovely when I sat here with Jane," Laura reflected, "and now you've made it even more beautiful."

* * *

Seated at the table, the candles softly lighting

our faces, we alternated between drifting conversation and quiet appreciation of the surroundings. We took our time with dinner, and then, as I was passing her the dessert, I glanced through the open door at the bedroom. Laura and I had never slept together there, preferring her place. Neither of us felt comfortable about her spending the night in the bed that had been Jane's and mine.

But I had a different idea.

"Do I remember correctly," I began, "that when your kids were younger, you did a lot of camping all over Israel?"

"Sure, you know that. Why do you ask?"

"Well, when you suggested the other day that you and I go camping, you meant cooking over a campfire, sleeping in a cramped tent, with grime and sweat, flies, and mosquitoes— the works, right?"

"That's right, camping."

"Well, I've been thinking about a different kind of camping. In a place more comfortable and with better amenities."

"And where might that place be?"

"Right over there on those two chaise lounges. Their backs fold down flat, and side by side, they make up into a double bed."

I paused.

"Jeff, dining together on this terrace has been lovely. But recalling the many times I sat out here with Jane—you and me sleeping together here would feel like an intrusion on those memories." She reached across the table and touched my hand. "I hope you understand."

* * *

An alternative thought came to mind when I glanced again into the bedroom.

"Laura, maybe, before clearing away the dishes, we could spend a few moments just lying together on the bed, fully clothed, and talk about how that feels."

Laura gave a faint nod. I took her hand and we walked inside. We kicked off our shoes and lay down facing each other on the bedspread, my head on my pillow, Laura's head on Jane's. We wrapped our arms around each other, and my cheek nestled against her forehead.

It had been about two and a half years since Jane had lain with me on that bed, and I felt warm and content there with Laura. What I didn't realize, though, was how uncomfortable she must have felt on Jane's half of the bed. It was only much later when she mentioned it to me that I realized how thoughtless I had been to suggest it.

Looking past Laura, Jane's computer screen stared at me from her bedside desk. I imagined Jane sitting there glued to the screen. She'd steal a look at Laura and me, then snap her head back to her computer, then steal another look.

"This is hard," I told Laura. "Jane's been gone for half a year, yet sometimes it feels like she's still here."

"I know."

"In fact, it feels that way right now, as though I can see her sitting right next to us."

"How does she look to you?" Laura asked.

"It's strange. One moment she's smiling, next her face is scrunched up with rage, and then she has tears rolling down her face."

"I'm guessing she would feel all those things," Laura answered.

I wished I could somehow console Jane, explain to her how pained I'd felt over the past few years, and how Laura had helped me through those difficult times.

Soon Laura and I got up, carried the dishes to the kitchen, washed them, and drove to her house.

| 31 |

Rainbow

"Welcome home to Ithaca, Professor Camhi" read the note taped to the front door of the white clapboard farmhouse. "What a long trip you've had! I'm out until dinnertime. Meanwhile, you know where your room is."

It was October 2015, nine months since Jane's death. Beside the door, a wooden sign read "Amazing Grace Bed and Breakfast." The current owner had bought the house from us thirty-three years earlier when we moved to Jerusalem, and she had later turned it into a B&B.

I had come back for a few days to attend the fiftieth anniversary celebration of Cornell's Department of Neurobiology and Behavior, where I had been a faculty member for fifteen years. As I was eager for my visit to reawaken memories, what better place for me to stay than in our old house?

I felt strangely disoriented, though, standing on the house's front stoop. Things looked different. Gone was Jane's big, fenced-in vegetable garden. Gone was the basketball hoop where Jeremy and I had sunk many a jump shot. Gone, and transformed into a parking area, was the terrace where I had grilled so many summer dinners and where we'd enjoyed them at our picnic table overlooking the deep valley.

Mostly, of course, gone was Jane. I had known that being alone there would be a challenge. Even more so, as I had booked not just any room but our former bedroom! I was hoping it would reawaken things forgotten and maybe bring me new insights.

* * *

With a sense of trepidation, I pushed open the front door and stepped into the living room.

Embers smoldering in the woodstove filled the room with a musky fragrance and fended off the early autumn chill. From the time Jeremy was seven or eight, he had tended that stove. As a teenager, he had split logs for firewood and learned the names and properties of all the tree types in our woods. I had little doubt that his early connection to trees and wood helped spark his profession as a fine woodworker.

I had my own connections to wood in that living room. Still standing was the floor-to-ceiling pine bookcase I had built along one wall to hold Jane's history and Judaism volumes. But the wooden object to which I had been, and remained, most attached, and which had sat in the now vacant alcove, was my baby grand Knabe piano. According to its serial number, it was manufactured a year after I was born, and we had grown up together. After separating from it when I went off to college, we were reunited in Cambridge and then remained so.

I wished my piano were there with me now; I imagined Jane calling out from a distant room, "Jeff, please play that one again" or walking by and blowing me a kiss.

Late in Jane's Alzheimer's, music had been one of the few ways I could reach her. I'd play the few songs she liked best again and again. Her favorite was "Over the Rainbow." Sometimes, she would sing a few of the words, even after she had all but stopped speaking.

Standing there in that Ithaca living room, I

remembered Jane's own remarkable entry into music. At the age of thirty-eight, she had decided to learn the cello, a decision that seemed to come out of nowhere; she played no other instrument. But the cello's deep resonance stirred her. She bought a good quality instrument and hired an excellent teacher who came to the house weekly, and there, in that Ithaca living room, beside my piano, Jane progressed from incipient squeaks to sustained vibratos that filled the whole house. Even when she was not playing, the cello had a presence, standing there upright in its black leather case. For inspiration, Jane also bought several recordings, especially those of cellist Jacqueline du Pré, whom she greatly admired. She practiced several hours a day, and within a year, she and three friends had formed a string quartet. They met every Wednesday evening, there in our living room, and played for hours. Jane had often claimed that Wednesday evenings were, for her, the high point of each week.

When we moved to Jerusalem, Jane helped form another string quartet that also assembled weekly in our living room. But at some point, she started playing wrong notes, getting the tempo wrong, or losing her place in the score.

It soon got worse.

One evening, after the members of her quartet had gone home, she returned her cello to its black leather case. She laid it to rest under my piano and never touched it again.

In a sense, Jane's illness had separated me from the piano as well; I hadn't played at all since her funeral and had kept both its keyboard cover and its lid permanently shut.

* * *

From the living room, I opened the door to the room I had booked. It looked very much as when it was our bedroom—the same deep crimson walls Jane had painted, the massive wood beams and exposed rafters she had stained dark brown, the off-white linoleum floor tiles I had laid, the walk-in clothes closet and shelves I had built, and the large picture window framing the valley's pastures and woods, now speckled with autumnal reds and yellows.

Of course, the furnishings were different now, and the owner seemed to liked clutter. Amid the jumble, my eyes fell upon a single wooden object positioned against the far wall—a beautiful music stand of rich, dark mahogany.

From its base sprang a sculpted male figure whose raised arms held the music tray on which lay a single piece of sheet music.

I crossed the room for a closer look.

Impossible!

"Over the Rainbow."

An original print, dated 1939. I lifted the sheet music, plopped down on the bed, and whispered the familiar lyrics as though I were speaking them to Jane.

* * *

Early the next morning, my laptop pinged. I clicked on an email from the dean of the science faculty at the Hebrew University. He was setting up a new program on science and art and wondered if I would join the organizing committee.

Art, I thought. Very nice, but what did I have to offer on that subject? Glancing over at the music stand, I had an idea. "Might music be part of your science and art program?" I responded.

"Why not?" he replied and asked what I had in mind.

I imagined there was plenty of musical talent on campus. But with everyone either buried in their research lab or studying for exams, there was little opportunity for this talent to emerge. Maybe it was time to bring it out into the open.

"Great idea," the dean replied. "Maybe make it a project of your open campus museum." I was, in fact, already planning that.

During the several days remaining in my Ithaca visit, I kept mulling over the idea of my developing a concert series at the university back home. I'd never done anything like that before. It seemed like a lot of work. But the more I thought about it, the more I liked it.

On my return to Jerusalem, I sent out emails to all students, faculty, and staff on the university's science campus, inviting anyone with performance experience in any musical genre to attend an organizational meeting and, if possible, to bring their instruments. Twenty-three students and faculty members showed up, many bearing instruments: violins, guitars, a cello, a trumpet, and two flutes. There were also pianists and singers. Several were accomplished musicians.

From then on, I slid into a role new to me, that of music director, and I found myself busy organizing a program of concerts, setting up and attending rehearsals, making suggestions, finding an appropriate venue on campus, and advertising the concerts.

The result was "The Musical Campus," a series of four concerts a year, each presenting a sequence of three or four different performers or groups—mostly science students and faculty—in a variety of musical genres. To my delight, each concert drew an audience of close to two hundred.

* * *

As plans for our first concert took shape, the musicians insisted that I also perform. But not having played since Jane's death, my fingers were badly out of condition.

Laura suggested that perhaps it was time to open my keyboard cover.

Days passed.

The challenge gnawed.

One morning, as the early sunlight shone through my living room windows, I sat down on Jane's Bargello-covered piano bench, took a look at her Annapurna photo propped up on the piano, and lifted the keyboard cover. Hesitantly, I pressed a few keys. Though my fingers felt stiff from disuse, they loosened up a little as

I played. I imagined that in the time left before our first concert, my fingers could be ready. But what about the rest of me?

At the opening concert, I sat next to Laura but stood to introduce each of the first three performances. I appeared last, playing what I had called "Improvisations on Great American Standards." I introduced each song with a brief comment, but I gave my last number a rather longer explanation. I first mentioned that it was written in the 1930s by Harold Arlen with lyrics by Yip Harburg and that, at the close of the twentieth century, it had been designated by the National Endowment for the Arts as the century's number-one popular song. I added that Judy Garland sang it in *The Wizard of Oz* and continued, "The song is, of course ..."

"'Over the Rainbow,'" a few people called out from the audience.

I went silent for a moment, half wanting to end the performance right there, say thank you, and slip away. But I held steady. "As some of you know, I lost my wife early this year after her long decline through Alzheimer's." I sensed a stillness in the room.

"Toward the end, when Jane had all but stopped speaking and had withdrawn into herself, I often played the piano for her. Music, and especially this, her favorite song, could still bring on her smile. Sometimes she would even sing out, appropriately, the words to the song's last five notes. Do you know those words?"

"Why, oh why, can't I?" a few people replied.

"Yes. This was her song. And I'd like to play it for you now."

Wanting the opening notes themselves to ascend and arch over the rainbow, I placed both my hands far to my left, very low on the keyboard, and turned each hand palm up. With both index fingers fully extended, I swept them up along almost the whole keyboard in a two-handed glissando, "Way up high," as the lyrics declare. Next, I found myself accompanying the descending scale of the song's main theme with thick chords, creating a somewhat dark sound. However, I then flipped that theme on its head by creating an ascending scale and decorated it with light, swirling inventions because, after all, over the rainbow can be a lovely place. A few more passes through the melody and I brought it to a conclusion by playing those five final ascending notes, "why, oh why, can't I?" singly and unaccompanied.

At first the audience didn't move. Then

applause. The dean clapped enthusiastically along with several of my colleagues, former graduate students, and our newly discovered campus musicians. Laura beamed.

I had been on a long journey.

I felt exhausted.

But at peace.

| 32 |

Stay or Go

I had planned to stay on in our home for at least a year after Jane's death to ease my way into whatever might come next. So far, ten months had passed. As Laura and I did not feel ready to cohabit, my choice was either to remain in the house or to look for someplace new for myself.

My decision was influenced by deep underground forces. According to a recent geological study, Israel was due for a major earthquake, perhaps the next day, or in ten years or more. Beneath the Jordan Valley, the study predicted, two opposing tectonic plates would rub shoulders, the ground above would lurch, and many buildings would come crashing down. Although mild earthquakes are fairly common in Israel, this one would be different. Buildings constructed before 1985, the year legal construction standards were upgraded, were deemed particularly vulnerable. My house dated from the 1920s.

Needing to find out whether the house was really unsafe, I arranged for an engineering evaluation.

* * *

A pair of highly recommended engineers showed up one morning. They checked every corner of the house, banging on walls, jumping on floors, and stomping on stairs to feel the resulting vibrations. Mostly, though, they pushed along the stone floors a little device on wheels that would sense whether the steel supports under the stones could bear a major quake.

Jane and I had selected the floor stones as part of our renovation before moving into the house. Just after signing the purchase papers, we had gone out to celebrate at the bar of the then new Plaza Hotel. The mottled, rose-colored stone flooring of the hotel's lobby and bar caught our eyes. As we sat sipping Martinis, we mused about how those stones would look in our new home and realized we just had to have that flooring. Once installed, it became the stage on which our lives were to play out for the next thirty years.

Now watching the engineers push their device along the floor, I felt like a patient undergoing an ultrasound, hoping it wouldn't uncover some deep, life-threatening ailment.

The test lasted two hours, after which one of the engineers stated: "You have a problem."

He explained that the steel rails supporting the floor were not attached to one another. In the case of an earthquake, each would move independently, the floors would be stressed, and they might well collapse. In fact, the whole house could collapse, he clarified.

As I envisioned all those pieces of mottled rose-colored stone coming apart, a tremor shot right through me. Surprisingly, though, a part of me was glad to receive this analysis—the part of me that felt ready to push forward and move out.

I decided that in two months' time—exactly one year after Jane's death—I would put the house on the market and let someone else deal with the structural renovations.

| 33 |

Trees

February 8, 2016, one year since Jane had died. Her first yahrzeit, the annual Jewish memorial service. Alon, Jeremy and family, and I, as well as those closest to us and to Jane, including Laura, visited her grave.

I arrived first and parked the car in exactly the same place I had the previous year. I walked the same route as I had then behind the stretcher bearing Jane.

It was different now, of course. There was Jane's lovely, newly installed, mottled rose-colored gravestone. Incised in the stone was the sentence "She saw the good in everyone." Jeremy, Alon, and I had agreed that this statement captured something essential about Jane.

I ran my forefinger through each of the engraved letters, feeling my way through each word, as though recomposing, reengraving, reconfirming it, knowing that this was one of the reasons why so many people loved and admired her. As I finished tracing the sentence, Jeremy, Alon, and others arrived. Jeremy said the appropriate prayers. Several others shared their feelings and stories about Jane, some amusing, others deeply moving. I felt warmed by the group that had, once again, collected around Jane.

* * *

The realtor had agreed not to advertise the sale of the house until after the yahrzeit, but I was not expecting, the very next morning, to see his sign already strung on my front gate.

The stone floors that had supported us, the white walls that had embraced us, the space we had filled with thirty years of living, all suddenly—shockingly—up for bids. But a consoling thought was quick to follow. Just as Jane remained in my memory and would travel with me wherever I went, so too would our house.

And so too would my memories of Golani. As I was soon moving, it was time for us to say goodbye too. After a lengthy search—not everyone wants a dog with only three working legs—he was finally adopted by a family with young children.

I looked again at the "For Sale" sign on the front gate. With one measure of sadness but another of impending freedom, I let the selling process commence.

Within two weeks, the house was sold.

* * *

I decided to lighten my load by renting another place instead of buying. This would leave me free to make more changes whenever the time seemed right.

Laura helped me scope out a suitable apartment, one in which she would be spending a considerable amount of time. We looked at only three apartments. The third was in a brand new building, centrally located, a short walk from Jerusalem's open market and from public transportation, and with private parking. The moment we entered that apartment, we were bathed in sunlight streaming through picture windows and a glass door opening onto a terrace nearly as large as the one off the bedroom of Jane's and my house.

Laura and I happily envisioned ourselves there, and I signed the rental agreement on the spot.

Laura helped me decide where to place things in the apartment. The piano went near the entrance to the living room, where Jane's Bargello seat cover was visible from every angle. The bookcase that had housed my seashell collection in my childhood bedroom fit neatly into my new bedroom, now holding books but topped by the large conch shell Laura had bought for me in China. The second bedroom, which became my study, was furnished by Jeremy, who made a beautiful desk, bookshelves, cabinets, and a wood-framed mirror.

It was Laura's idea to relocate from the house's terrace garden all of Jane's trees, shrubs, and flowers in planters—to the new apartment's terrace.

We arranged for a crane to lift all the planters from the house and hoist them onto the apartment's terrace. When all was in order and the workers left, we walked around the transported plants, thankful that they had all survived the journey.

"It will be like having a little bit of Jane here," Laura commented.

I reached out and squeezed her hand.

I was looking particularly at the trees, recalling how small they had been when Jane had planted them.

"These trees," I whispered. "All the time Jane was shrinking, they just kept right on growing."

Laura thought about that and then responded, "Just like someone I know."